ISBN: 1492937274
ISBN 13: 9781492937272

TABLE OF CONTENTS

PART I

DIET, EXERCISE,
SEE ME IN SIX MONTHS

MY NAME IS PAUL RAMIREZ, AND MY LIFE AND HEALTH HAVE BEEN TRANS-FORMED BY DR. DAVE AND CLAYTON TOTAL HEALTH.

I just turned fifty-five; have an adult, married daughter with a loving husband and three lovely children; have a beautiful girlfriend; have an enviable career; and live in one of the world's great cities.

I have a lot to live for.

I'd noticed over the past few years that I'd spent more time seeing the doctor, visiting hospitalized friends and relatives—some of whom recovered, some of whom didn't—and viewing those relentless ads telling me to "ask my doctor."

I'd believed that my diet was fine, that my fitness was fine, and that, for a man in my early/mid- 50s, I was fine.

This past Christmas, my son-in-law's dad died. And my son-in-law was angry that the choices his father had made, and had refused to make, had cost him his life and his grandchildren's opportunity to know and love their grandfather.

I believe his death was untimely and altogether preventable.

Not long after, I met with Dr. Dave—not because I was sick, but because my new girlfriend wanted me to provide her with a clean bill of my sexual health. During that consultation, Dave noted that my blood pressure was steadily increasing and asked if I was aware of the impact that it would have on my overall, and sexual, health.

He asked me what I intended to do about it and recommended that we take a closer look, ordering comprehensive blood analyses.

My STD results came back clean but my heart and fitness results did not. Those items most critical to wellness: blood pressure, CRP, cholesterol, and triglycerides, were high at worst, and at best, on the margin.

I was not fine.

This was my "Oh shit!" moment.

Dave explained my options: continue to live my "fine" lifestyle and become dependent on every drug the ads tell me to ask my doctor about, or improve my health by dedicating myself to a lifestyle of sensible diet and fitness.

My choice was simple and clear, and it is one that I encourage every man in my condition to make.

Dave offers a medically supervised diet and fitness program. Its impact is supported by scientific evidence, common sense, and the testimony of those who have adopted it.

In 100 days I've lost ten pounds and shifted flab to muscle. I sleep better, worry less, and have improved my sexual virility and self-image.

HERE ARE THE FACTS AND DATA:

- My CRP[1] has declined 61%, from high risk to normal.

- My total cholesterol has declined 12%, from borderline to desirable.

- My "bad" cholesterol has declined 18%, from desirable to optimal.

---

1 CRP is a measure of total body inflammation. High CRP levels are associated with a greater risk of heart attack or stroke.

- My triglycerides dropped by half, from nearly 300 to under 150.

- My Real LDL size pattern has fundamentally shifted from small/dense to large/buoyant—from more risk to less risk.

- My blood pressure has come down from the 140/90 range to a more respectable 120/85.

- I receive several "wows" daily from friends, family, colleagues and, most importantly, that new girlfriend.

THESE STELLAR CHANGES ARE THE RESULT OF THREE THINGS:

1) Four days of medically supervised cross-training, designed and led by Dr. Dave and his colleagues. This is a man who walks the talk and has channeled his academic, professional, and personal experience into transforming lives without pharmaceutical intervention.

2) Seven days a week of eating pure, fresh food according to a simple rule: if it existed a million years ago, eat it; if it didn't, don't.

3) Collaborating with a growing community of men who are committed to living long, healthful, and virile lives.

I encourage you to do your homework. Study the facts. Talk to the charter members of Clayton MD Total Health about their experience with diet, fitness, and flushing their meds.

Then ask your doctor about what you can do. Just make sure his name is Dr. Dave.

I still have work to do—my blood pressure and triglycerides remain borderline and I am motivated to move those metrics next. I am confident that in the next 100 days those wild beasts, too, will be tamed. I, my new mates at Clayton MD Total Health, and Dr. Dave will hold me accountable to that!

INTRODUCTION

by Dr. Dave Clayton

PAUL'S PROBLEMS ARE HARDLY UNIQUE. In fact, chronic disease has become an accepted part of the aging process. If you are over sixty and not on any medication you are in the minority. One in two adults of any age has at least one chronic medical problem and by the time we're over sixty nearly 90% of people are on at least one medication daily. In addition, a staggering one-third of adults over sixty take five or more medications daily. Most of these medications are for the trifecta of modern living: diabetes, high blood pressure, and high cholesterol. Paul's no exception—he's in the majority.

These numbers are staggering, but we've become jaded to stats like these as chronic disease becomes the new normal. You've certainly heard by now that these diseases and others are a result of poor diet and lack of exercise. Many of us are familiar with the constant refrain from physicians that we've all got to eat better and exercise more. Every time you go in for an office visit you hear the same thing, yet how often does this goading translate into real improvement in your health?

For over fifteen years I was one of those doctors prescribing the familiar "diet, exercise, see me in six months." For the most part, my advice was in vain. My patients would swear up and down that they were trying their hardest but the blood pressure would keep going up, along with the cholesterol and the blood sugars. Older patients who were diligently taking calcium and vitamin D would still end up with osteoporosis. My most unlucky patients would start to lose their memories and I would have little to offer them in terms of solace or drugs. We would simply accept the fact that they must be genetically predisposed to getting sick or that this was just an inevitable part of aging.

JUST BLAME IT ON YOUR PARENTS

Most of my patients were legitimately trying. They would read books on nutrition and watch the news closely for the latest health updates. They would eat healthy and walk three times a week for exercise just like their last doctor advised. Most were taking at least a few supplements and sometimes as many as ten or more per day. Hardly anyone in my practice was an unabashed couch potato with a bag of Doritos by his side—most were trying to do everything that their doctors were telling them to do. But it wasn't helping.

When such lifestyle changes didn't work we would invariably chalk up poor health to family history or genetics. Genetics is not only a popular scapegoat for health problems but also the favorite pursuit of those looking for solutions. You can't turn on the television or open the newspaper without learning about the newest breakthrough in genetics. It is as though personalized medicine and genomics will somehow solve our problems the same way a great suit can hide our curves. For less than $100 you can even have your genes tested without ever having to leave your home. With all this public focus it is hard to fault anyone for blaming disease on parents or genetics—how could chronic disease be within our control? It must be something buried in our genetics that makes us somehow prone to eat ice cream and put on weight. Damn genetics!

But how important is family history really? The numbers speak for themselves: if 90% of people over sixty are on medication and half of all adults of any age have high cholesterol, high blood pressure, or diabetes, then the chances are pretty good that you've got a family history of something. After all, who in the U.S. doesn't have a family history of chronic disease? Only a lucky few of us will have two perfectly healthy parents, not to mention siblings, grandparents, or aunts and uncles. You don't have to look far down the branches of a family tree to find more than a bit of chronic disease.

Statistically, this argument that we are helpless to our genetics just doesn't hold water. Sure, a few of us may be genetically more or less prone to certain diseases, but this simply makes diet and exercise all the more important. The more the deck is stacked against you, the better you need to play your hand.

WELCOME TO MIDLIFE, DOC!

The turning point for me was when I hit my midlife crisis two decades too early. I've always been an active person, working out several times a week and eating right. If my weight creeps up a few pounds, I rein in my diet until I'm back in range again. So it came as quite a shock to me when I began to see my blood pressure creep up to the borderline range more and more often. Furthermore, my LDL cholesterol was nearly 140, with my total cholesterol over 230. I couldn't believe it—I was eating a healthy, balanced diet, working out nearly every day, and I was in nearly the best shape of my life. Yet despite all this hard work and conscientious eating, I was probably going to need medication for both my blood pressure and my cholesterol before I hit forty.

IT'S HARDER THAN IT LOOKS

That is when it dawned on me that "diet and exercise" is harder than it looks. I've lectured my patients for years on how they should eat better and exercise more, but if even a physician and certified health nut can't succeed with diet and exercise, then who can? How could I possibly expect my patients to be able to accomplish with diet and exercise what I couldn't? I soon found out that I wasn't alone in my dilemma; nearly every physician with whom I worked at the time was taking one or more medications for common metabolic conditions.

I could have chalked it up to family history; my mother has high cholesterol and my father has high blood pressure. But I was convinced that my healthy living would protect me from such heritage and was determined not to give in so easily. So after fifteen years of practicing medicine the old-fashioned way, I threw the rule book out the door and tried to understand why so many of my patients were unable to see real results with traditional diet and exercise. I became a voracious student of nutrition as it relates to metabolic diseases. I pored over research journals, read textbooks, and attended scientific sessions. What I learned caused me to change my thinking about how to define "diet and exercise". What I learned changed my life and my health, and transformed the way that I treat my patients.

DIGGING FOR TREASURE AND FINDING IT

I found that buried among the millions of research papers in the National Institutes of Health database are a number of truly remarkable studies that demonstrate how our diet affects our health. I focused on those studies where there was a compelling correlation between specific dietary and physical actions and the incidence and severity of chronic disease. As I did my research, a stunning conclusion emerged: almost all of the chronic diseases we associate with aging can be prevented, treated, or cured by adopting specific dietary and exercise strategies. Not only that, but in many cases, the improvement actually exceeds that achieved with medications, and without all the side effects.

As a physician I was completely amazed to learn how amenable certain conditions are to diet and exercise. For example, as you'll read in a later chapter, diet and exercise can lower blood pressure by up to thirty points or more (for example, from 150/90 to 120/80). This is a shocking reduction, especially when you compare it to the paltry nine point reduction you would get with the maximum dose of a leading branded blood pressure medication. In fact, it might take three or more drugs to get the same blood pressure lowering as you could get with diet and exercise. In addition, these drugs have consequences; common side effects include sexual dysfunction, fatigue, and dizziness. Before you know it, you need another drug or two just to fix the side effects of the first three.

High cholesterol is another one that is entirely fixable with diet and exercise. Studies show that cholesterol can be lowered by 30% or more with diet and exercise alone. This is about what you would expect from a starting dose of any of the statin-class cholesterol medications. The only difference is that statins might cause muscle cramps and have been associated with an increased risk of diabetes and memory loss. I can promise you that eating healthy won't have any of those side effects and could lower your cholesterol by more than even a statin could. If we add on some natural dietary supplements, the cholesterol-lowering is even more dramatic—I've seen reductions in cholesterol approaching 50% without using any medication at all.

Treating conditions like blood pressure, diabetes, and high cholesterol with diet and exercise gives us results over just weeks to months. But the successes don't stop there. Numerous studies have shown that diet and exercise are as good as, or better than, medications for heart disease, heart failure, stroke, Alzheimer's disease, and osteoporosis, among others. *In fact, Alzheimer's disease is virtually untreatable by medications but can be almost entirely prevented with diet and exercise.*

Data like these are just the tip of the iceberg. We're all going to get older, but we don't have to get sicker. Most, if not all, of the age-related conditions I used to treat with medications could be treated just as well or better with diet and exercise. I became convinced that treating my patients with medications and sending them off on their own to figure out diet and exercise was missing the forest for the trees.

MY SOLUTION

That's where this book comes in. The vast preponderance of medical research suggests that most (if not all) of the chronic diseases associated with aging are a result of our diet. Interestingly, there is a common theme among most nutrition research: the foods that have been proven to heal are those on which we evolved. For millions of years we adapted to our environment and our diet, and it was only in the past few thousand years that this diet began to change. Our diet today—even a healthy diet—is vastly different from that of our ancestors. Over 70% of the calories in even a healthy modern diet come from foods that simply didn't exist even a few thousand years ago. As we learn more about the foods that cause disease and the foods that cure, it becomes clear that our evolutionary diet is the foundation of good health. One rule—if it wasn't around a million years ago, don't eat it—explains why diets as different as vegetarian and Atkins can both improve your health, and explains the lower incidence of chronic diseases in cultures as different as the Mediterranean and Asia. We don't need to figure out a healthy diet; nature has provided the rules for us already.

But staying true to our evolutionary diet is not the entire solution. If that were true we could live forever on a diet of coconuts and rib-eye steaks. Beyond demonstrating the links between natural foods and health, modern research also tells us why certain foods have the ability to cure disease. In search of the health tips that truly make a difference in our health, I found that the 80/20 rule applies in nutrition the same way it applies elsewhere in life. About 80% of the benefit from a healthy diet accrues from only a handful of important tips. These tips, all consistent with the principles of our evolutionary diet, are ones that most of us have already heard but that few of us ever put into practice.

I've sorted through thousands of research articles, ranging from the first studies on cholesterol published back in the 1920s all the way to the latest research on fish oil and cancer. From them I have identified the four diet tips that, when done poorly or not at all, account for the bulk of problems of chronic disease and aging. These four diet tips I put into the form of Challenges, which give you the opportunity to do what so few people ever do—put your knowledge and intentions into real actions and see the results.

THE PROOF

When I first started putting this project together, I was my own first subject. I took the diet Challenges one at a time, learning new recipes and adopting new foods step by step. The results were exactly as I had hoped; my LDL cholesterol dropped by over 40% without medication, and my blood pressure came down to a totally reasonable 110/80. Despite the fact that I had a family history of high blood pressure and high cholesterol, I'd cured them both in less than two months with this program.

I then started to make these recommendations to my patients. One by one, I started to see dramatic results. Literally every single person who followed this plan saw some improvement in their numbers. Like Paul, those who put the most effort into following my recommendations and who began a vigorous exercise program saw the most benefit, lowering their doses of medications or dropping them altogether. You'll read their stories as you go through the book.

One of the best things about this strategy is that it isn't experimental. It's not some new theory that is yet to be proven; nor is it made up out of thin air. In fact, this plan is exactly the opposite. Everything in this program has been proven in clinical trials to be scientifically sound. This plan is about putting the most important scientific evidence on diet, nutrition, and exercise into an actionable program that gets you beyond reading and into doing and seeing results.

After nearly two years of putting this program into practice among my patients, I realized that they needed more than my advice and encouragement every few months during their scheduled office visits. I started with a handful of pioneering patients who were willing to put their overall health and fitness in my hands. Over the course of an entire year, we worked out together three days a week, discussing nutrition, going over diet logs, and sharing recipes. Our workouts focused on all the important goals that most people miss in their workouts: cardio, weight training, balance, core strength and stability, and agility. Their results were astounding. They started dropping medications one after another. Their numbers improved dramatically, with significant reductions in blood sugars, blood pressure, and other metrics. Even better, my guys started moving better. They reported better balance, fewer falls, and less aches and pains. It didn't take long for me to realize that this was exactly what my patients needed to take charge of their health and start living better every single day.

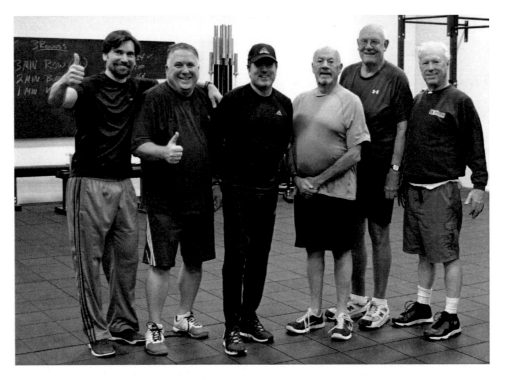

Thus, with the support of my family and this core group of die-hard patients, Clayton MD Total Health was born. I left the traditional practice of medicine in order to create a comprehensive health center, a "club" based on the singular purpose of helping people get healthy, stay healthy, and live a long time, free of disease, using the principles outlined in this book. Clayton MD Total Health is designed from the ground up to provide you with all the resources you need to get healthy and stay healthy, no matter your age. I'll give you the tools—all you have to do is show up and have fun. The results will be better than you could ever imagine.

HOW TO USE THIS BOOK

You don't have to be a member of my health club to see results with this book, but it helps. If you must exercise on your own, be sure to read my comments on exercise and put them to use in your own program.

The first half of the book is an introduction to the concept of an evolutionary hunter-gatherer diet. Here I give you the basic fundamentals of our native diet and explain the links between modern foods and disease. This is the foundation for the second part of the book where you will find the Challenges.

The Challenges are where the rubber meets the road. In order to truly start turning back the clock on the aging process, you must first master the evolutionary diet. With this under your now-looser belt you will turn your attention to the last four Challenges. These will push your knowledge of nutrition to a new level, and you'll finally get—really get—why basic lessons like "eat more fiber" are so important to your health. You'll learn why these tips work and why most people get them wrong. More importantly, you'll learn how you can get them right and see a dramatic improvement in your health in the process. You will understand the difference between "diets" and a sustainable lifestyle focused on quality of life.

I recommend spending at least two to four weeks or more on each Challenge. It will take you that long to develop new habits and break the old ones. Along the way you will learn new recipes, experiment with new foods, and keep track of your progress. I highly recommend that you keep a log of your food intake, home blood pressure readings, and home blood sugar readings, if applicable.

There are a number of metrics that I usually follow in my office that I encourage you to follow as well. You should see improvements in some or all of the following within the first ninety days:

- Blood pressure

- Cholesterol, including LDL, HDL, triglycerides, LDL particle size, and LDL particle number

- Hemoglobin A1c (a blood test that represents the average blood sugar over the past three months), fasting blood sugar, and insulin levels

- C-reactive protein (a measure of total body inflammation, associated with everything from heart disease to asthma and arthritis)

- Body weight

- Percent body fat

- Waist and hip measurements

If you are on medications for cholesterol, diabetes, or blood pressure, I expect you to be able to get results from this program equivalent to or better than what you are getting from your medications. You will be healthier and require fewer medications. No more worrisome side effects and no more adding medications with every year. Instead, we'll be able to start reducing or eliminating the medications and I can assure you that you will feel younger and more energetic than you have in years.

Sound good? I thought so. Now let's get started!

SAFETY FIRST. *This program is specifically designed to improve your health and reduce your need for certain medications. Because of its effectiveness you should be careful to monitor your blood pressure, and if applicable, your blood sugars, regularly once you start. Do not stop or lower the dose of any of your medications without first checking with your doctor. Also, you should check with your doctor before beginning any vigorous exercise program.*

BEFORE WE BEGIN, I'D LIKE TO GIVE YOU SOME ADVICE. Change is hard. You may have to change your lifestyle pretty dramatically in order to get off and stay off medications. A friend once told me, "If it was easy, everyone would be doing it." He was right–just taking Lipitor or any other drug is the easy way out, and everyone *is* doing it. Seventy million people are on cholesterol medications, which is a number equivalent to one out of every four Americans.

So expect the change to be hard, but also expect to be successful. Once you adopt your new healthy habits, you will find them to be second nature. You will feel better and you will feel good about it. I know, because I've been there myself. I got through it, my patients have gotten through it, and so will you. So let's start with a few very basic rules to live by:

THE NINE COMMANDMENTS

#1: NEVER EAT WHEN YOU ARE HUNGRY. Having any control over your diet is nearly impossible if you are starving. The craving for pizza, crackers, cookies, or even a tortilla or slice of bread can become overwhelming for anyone on an empty stomach. So don't let yourself get there. Don't skip meals and instead try to eat frequently during the day. You will make wiser choices if you have your meal before you become hungry, when your mind is clear and you are in control. Ideally, you should be trying for about 200–300 calories every 2–3 hours. Another benefit of this strategy is that you will feel more energetic and avoid the ups and downs of volatile sugar and insulin levels throughout your day.

#2: DON'T EAT FREE FOOD. Free food is sure to be a metabolic disaster. When was the last time you put serious thought into the food you brought for colleagues at a meeting or friends at a party? Chances are you brought cupcakes, sandwiches, or pizza and probably went for the cheaper rather than the healthier option. When someone else hosts the meeting or party, keep your hands to yourself and be ready with some food of your own. Saving money just isn't worth it.

#3: BE PREPARED. If you aren't thinking ahead, you're going to get hungry. Plan your meals ahead of time. When you are winding down at the end of the day, take a few minutes to think about the next day. What will you cook at home; what will you snack on? If you are eating out, where will you go? What will you buy? Pack some nuts to snack on or some leftovers from the day before. If you're going to be in a rush tomorrow morning, make breakfast the night before and take it on the go. Think about what restaurants you might stop at for lunch and what you'll order. If the refrigerator is bare, put together a shopping list. When you are planning your meals and snacks ahead of time you are more likely to make smart, conscious decisions about nutrition.

#4: LEARN A NEW WAY OF COOKING. When we adopt a new diet, the natural first step is to get rid of all the "bad" foods. Unfortunately, this means taking away foods without much thought going into what will replace them. This leaves us with a plate half-empty and our stomachs craving for more. We skip meals, get hungry, get frustrated, and finally revert to our old ways. A healthy lifestyle is not about deprivation but learning how to fill your plate with delicious and nutritious foods. Don't expect to get comfortable with this overnight without putting in some effort. You will have to learn how to turn vegetables into something other than salad and venture beyond red meat for other protein sources. There are literally millions of great recipes out there that are consistent with good nutrition. I'll give you some recipes to get you started and show you where to find more. Enjoy the process of finding recipes; challenge yourself to get creative.

#5: TAKE CONTROL OF YOUR OWN HEALTH. If only I had a nickel for every time I heard from one of my patients that he can't change his diet because his [kids, spouse, girlfriend, etc.] wouldn't go for it. It is easy to give up control of your diet to someone else, and it conveniently absolves you of any responsibility for your own choices—"My kids will only eat pizza so I'm going to have to eat pizza." Don't let this happen to you. You are in control of your own health. Make conscious decisions and don't let someone else's views on health and nutrition affect yours.

#6: GET YOUR FAMILY ON BOARD. It is really hard to stick to a new diet if everyone else in the house is doing things the old way (the way that got you onto your medication in the first place). Let your loved ones know that this is for your health, that it is what your doctor recommended, that it is to reduce your likelihood of having a stroke or a heart attack, and that it is to get you healthier so you will be around longer. If you are clear and unwavering about what you are doing, they will come around in time.

#7: COMMIT THE TIME THAT IT TAKES TO MAKE THE CHANGE. Perhaps the most common complaint I hear in the office is "I don't have time for [exercise, cooking, eating healthy, etc.]." I know you're busy—it's tough raising a family, maintaining a marriage, and having a career. Even in retirement, somehow the schedule still fills up with plenty of odds and ends. It's pretty easy to fill a day and pretty easy to let your health start to slide along the way. This isn't about *having* the time or *finding* the time to exercise and eat right—it's about *making* the time.

I find that most people can make the time in a week to exercise and cook, especially if we make it fun and not a chore. That's the reason I have made this program as fun as possible. Commit at least five hours a week to taking care of yourself. That's 3–4 hours of exercise and 1–2 hours of food prep every week—at a minimum. Decide ahead of time when those hours will be, block them off, and protect them with your life. If your boss demanded that you spend one hour each day attending a company-wide meeting, or your daughter needed to be picked up each day from soccer, you'd make time to do it, wouldn't you? Turn off your cell phone, ignore distractions, and give yourself the time you need to take care of yourself. Trust me, everyone will still be there when you get back from the gym.

#8: ACCEPT THAT IT WILL BE DIFFICULT—AT FIRST. Give yourself the time to adapt to a new way of living. It takes about a month or two for change to stick, which is one reason to slow down and take one challenge at a time as you go through this book. Put in the time to learn the new ways of eating and you will find that the second and third months go a lot easier. By then it should be second nature.

#9: EXPECT RESISTANCE. From everyone. Even those who love you. I hate to say it, but this plan really only works for one person...you. You're probably pretty busy ("I don't have time to exercise..."), and the reason you're so busy is that you're running around nonstop for everyone else. Taking time for yourself, time that you let slip as a priority years ago, means taking time away from what you are doing for everyone around you. It's five hours per week not at work, not at home with the family, not fixing the car. You need to be consistent and keep this time on the calendar each week. Avoid the temptation to go back to old habits. Expect some resistance and you'll be better able to deal with it when it comes. Trust me—they will come around once they see you are serious about what you are doing—and all of you start to see the results.

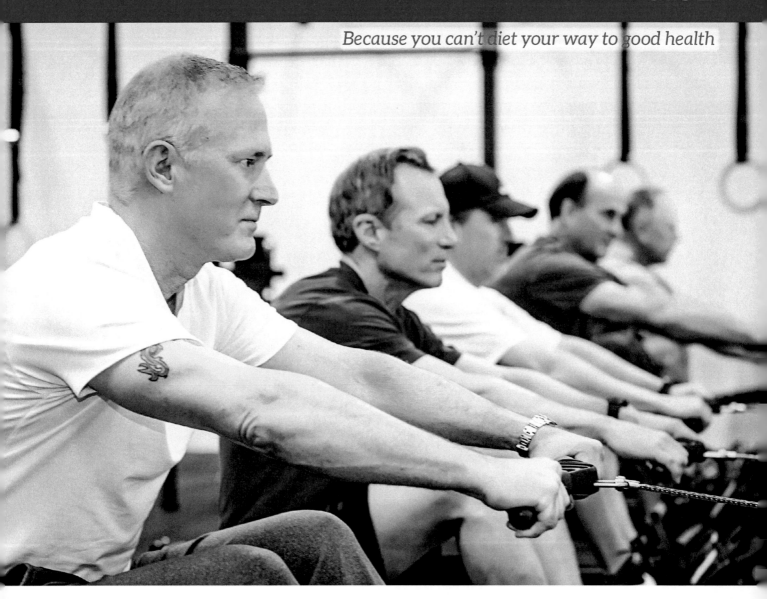

EXERCISE

Because you can't diet your way to good health

MANY OF MY PATIENTS HAD BEEN WALKING, HIKING, GOING TO THE GYM, OR PLAYING TENNIS AND GOLF BEFORE THEY MET ME. Unfortunately, despite all this activity, few of these people were getting slimmer, stronger, or taking fewer medications.

The problem is that we often confuse *activity* with *exercise*. Activity is being up and around, staying mobile and active. I would call a leisurely game of tennis or golf, walking, or hiking an *activity* rather than exercise. In contrast, *exercise* is pushing the limits of your physical activity in order to maintain or increase your functional ability.

Vigorous exercise has incredible benefits. Exercise increases lean muscle mass, reduces body fat, increases insulin sensitivity, lowers blood pressure, increases good HDL cholesterol, increases bone density, and increases men's testosterone levels. Even more importantly, exercise has been associated with an improved lifespan and a decreased risk of Alzheimer's disease and dementia. Translation: exercise helps you live a long time, free of disease, with a better quality of life on as few medications as possible.

Exercise is often tough medicine to take. Despite the amazing impact exercise has on our health, we are somehow inclined to eschew it whenever possible. We are inherently lazy, parking close to the mall and preferring the elevator over the stairs. Perhaps it is a throwback to the days when exercise was about survival (e.g., running from lions, building shelter, finding food). With so much activity dedicated to the basics of survival it is no wonder that we evolved to take advantage of any rest we could get.

With our natural proclivity toward inactivity, even if we do show up for a workout we may find it hard to really exert ourselves. We space out on the treadmill or the elliptical, then after 20–30 minutes we get off, having barely broken a sweat. Why? Because exercise can be boring, and it's hard, and the results are uncertain and in the future while the pain and boredom are right there in the present.

Furthermore, our bodies are extremely efficient. Try walking a mile the first time and you might have to stop three times. In a few months you'll be able to walk the entire mile without losing your breath or breaking a sweat. Your hip flexors, quadriceps, hamstrings, and calf muscles will adapt to the challenge of walking, getting stronger in all the areas that are needed for that one particular task. Once your body adapts, the walk becomes easier. This may be one reason that many of my patients persist with the same routine over and over again–walking the same route, biking the same neighborhood, taking the same hikes. Unfortunately, the ease suggests that the body has completely adapted to that routine. With the adaptation and the ease go the results. Forget about making any progress if your exercise routine is all about walking in circles.

Staying in your comfort zone, performing the same exercise day after day, is the surest way to minimize your returns. You burn fewer calories, are less engaged mentally, and limit the extent to which your muscles develop. Besides, how much fun is it anyway? You are doing the same thing day after day.

In order to get the most out of your efforts to improve your health without medications, you absolutely *must* engage in vigorous exercise. It doesn't matter what age you are –even in your sixties, seventies, and beyond, you can push yourself to new limits every week. Before you put on your track shoes and get started, I'll explain how to get the maximum results from your workouts:

MEASURE EVERYTHING. You can't improve it if you can't measure it. It's important to keep track of your progress and continually benchmark yourself against past accomplishments. Keep a journal handy and jot down important metrics such as the amount of weight lifted, time spent, or repetitions completed. This way you can go back anytime to see where you are relative to where you've been.

INCREASE THE INTENSITY. Did you row 400 meters in two and a half minutes today? Let's try for two minutes and twenty-five seconds tomorrow. When you push for new records, you start to see significant benefits from exercise. Your heart rate increases, your stride lengthens, and you recruit additional muscle fibers. You begin to burn more calories and improve your insulin sensitivity. What was once leisurely has become purposeful.

MIX IT UP. Remember how I told you that your body adapts to exercise? Don't let that happen to you. Get out there and run, row, climb ropes, flip tires, pull sleds, and lift weights. If you never do the same thing twice in a row you'll stay mentally engaged and physically challenged.

KEEP IT SAFE. Remember that you're a grownup looking to get healthy and stay healthy, not a professional athlete or an Olympic lifter. Train with people like you and keep to a pace that works. Protect your joints and know what you are doing before you do it. Working out with a trainer in a supervised group setting is ideal for safely pushing limits. And remember to always get clearance from your doctor or doctors before starting any exercise program.

SET GOALS. You can't just show up for exercise nor do it because you have to. You have to want to. Think about throwing away that bottle of pills or what it would feel like to be able to crank out a dozen perfect push-ups. Think about wanting to be able to always pick up your children, or your grandchildren, without pain, and teach them your favorite sport. Or simply picture yourself, fit and healthy, at age ninety-five, still driving yourself, hosting parties, and enjoying your life. That's the vision that will keep you focused and on the path to success.

HAVE FUN. Working out shouldn't be work. You socialize over lunch or at the golf course, so why not over a good workout? Fitness is a team sport, so make it a social occasion that you look forward to every day.

That's all for my introductory words of advice and encouragement. Now it's time to roll up our sleeves and start digging into the evolutionary diet that is the very foundation of good health.

PART II

THE EVOLUTIONARY DIET

EVOLUTION AND HEALTH

IF THERE IS ONE THING THAT WILL GET YOU THINKING ABOUT WHAT YOU PUT IN YOUR BODY, IT IS WATCHING A CHILD GROW. When my son turned ten months old I caught myself marveling at how much he'd grown since birth, quadrupling in size from six to twenty-four pounds. It then dawned on me that those extra eighteen pounds he didn't have at birth had come from only one place: the food that he eats. Somehow he had converted all that formula, breast milk, and mashed veggies into eighteen pounds of brain, flesh, and bone. He truly is what he eats. As adults, we often forget that the same holds true for us.

We often think of our bodies as static organisms; we eat for fuel, burn what we need, store what we can, and poop out the rest. Calories in, calories out. This simplistic view is quite far from the truth. The cells in our bodies turn over constantly—the cells in your gut last only a few days while your entire liver is reborn every 1–2 years. Aside from a few nerve cells that last in perpetuity, your body is in a state of constant regeneration.

With this in mind it becomes clear that what we eat is an important determinant of our health. Every cell and biological process in our body relies on the food we ingest to function correctly. Electrolytes such as sodium, potassium, and calcium pass back and forth through cell membranes, signaling everything from a light touch to a heartbeat. Fats are incorporated into cellular membranes to form the very structure of our tissues, yet they are also critical components of important pathways, signaling inflammation throughout the body. Moreover, fats compose the protective boundaries of cells in the central nervous system, ensuring that the brain, spinal cord, and eyes function perfectly. Proteins form both the muscles in our bodies and the myriad enzymes that facilitate chemical reactions for everything from digesting food to attacking invading organisms. Everything we ingest contributes to our functioning well or poorly.

What happens if we do not supply our body with the essential nutrients that we need? We have a word for what happens when our biological systems start to malfunction, and that word is "disease." Too much inflammation and we get heart disease, arthritis, or asthma. Imbalances of sodium, potassium, or calcium lead to high blood pressure, heart attacks, or bone fractures. A full 70% or more of the chronic diseases we physicians see every day can be traced back to nutrition.

Figuring out exactly the right balance of nutrients sometimes feels like an impossible task. It seems as though every day the media present us with another headline "Must Know" fact about the importance of something or the danger of something else. There is a similarly overwhelming trove of clinical research dissecting the normal functioning of the human body and the basis for disease. It would take a lifetime of study to understand the nuances of human nutrition and the perfect balance of nutrients for optimal health and longevity.

Thankfully there is an easier way to look at things, and that is through the lens of evolution. Through this lens, the nutritional landscape instantly becomes clearer as we understand in the most basic terms how nutrition affects our health.

YOU'VE BEEN SELECTED

In evolutionary terms, you and I are survivors. We have survived through millions of years of evolutionary pressure–i.e., natural selection–to arrive here on this planet today.

What is "natural selection"? Natural selection is the theory that, over time, a population will come to represent the best genetic fit for the environment. In any given population some people will naturally be more genetically suited to their surroundings. These lucky few will out-procreate the less fortunate and eventually will make up nearly the entire population.

Natural selection favors genetic traits that confer a survival benefit. When our environment is relatively stable, the population comes to represent the best overall genetic fit for that environment. This process of natural selection takes generations and occurs over hundreds of thousands or millions of years, eventually reaching equilibrium. If the environment changes, the population becomes a poor fit for the new environment and natural selection again starts to work, moving the genetic makeup of the population to a new norm in harmony with the new environment.

Mankind is no stranger to evolution and natural selection; in fact, evolution is taught in nearly every grade school biology class. The evidence of our adapting to our environment is readily apparent. We can look at our sharp incisors for biting and molars for crushing and chewing, opposable thumbs for grasping and fists for pounding, and melanin, which protects our skin from ultraviolet rays. Those adaptations are ones that we take for granted today and that most of us would readily acknowledge as being consistent with evolutionary adaptation. Isn't it logical that we would have developed the digestive tract and metabolic pathways for our native environment as well? Our bodies adapted to our environment and the challenges we faced in terms of nutrition, climate, and food availability. Our environment evolved slowly and our bodies evolved at the same pace—an evolutionary pace, measured in hundreds of thousands and millions of years. *Millions.*

We humans have been around for anywhere from 2.5 to 7 million years, depending on how many apes you want to include in our lineage. Our diet has changed little over this time, and what changes have occurred came millions of years apart.

Our earliest ancestors, much like modern apes, foraged for insects and plants. Later we would add meat to the diet, first by scavenging, then by hunting and fishing. For most of the past several million years (over 99.996% to be exact) we have had the exact same foods to choose from: nuts, seeds, fruits, vegetables, meat, and fish. There wasn't much else around to eat and certainly nothing we could consume with only our bare hands, sticks, and rudimentary stone tools. We were first gatherers, then hunter-gatherers. When all the food in a region was consumed we would simply pack our bags and head off in search of more. For millions of years our ancestors survived and flourished by living off wild plants and animals.

During these millions of years our bodies had plenty of time to adapt to their surroundings. The seasons changed, ice ages came and went, but the basic ingredients found in nature did not change one bit—our selections remained limited to nuts, seeds, fruits, vegetables, meat, and fish. These ingredients provided the materials for everything from an eyelash down to our very DNA. The role of each organ, from our brains and nervous systems to our joints, hearts, and kidneys, was established in response to millions of years of adaptation to our natural environment. You and I survived millions of years of evolution as foragers, gatherers, and hunter-gatherers to arrive here today.

In a world where the basic food groups have never changed, the body has the ability to adapt over time. It takes thousands to millions of years to see evolutionary change. During that time, humans who could not handle the long winters or who could not digest meat and vegetables would naturally not survive as well as those who could. Only the best adapted of our ancestors would survive thousands of generations of natural selection to populate the Earth. Our ancestors, yours and mine, were by their very definition the most highly adapted to the hunter-gatherer diet.

SURE, I CAN IMPROVE ON THAT

Approximately 10,000 years ago this paradigm—the environment that we had evolved to fit—changed dramatically. Was it an ice age, a meteor striking the Earth, or some other natural disaster? Nope. Ten thousand years ago, one of our intrepid ancestors got tired of looking for food and had the inspired idea of planting a row of crops. Since then life has never been the same.

Paradoxically, the very same advancement that allowed us to evolve socially beyond our hunter-gatherer roots is the same one that has eventually led to chronic disease today. After millions of years we stopped wandering the Earth and began to settle around stable plots of land that could be farmed for a steady stream of food. We figured out how to turn grains, inedible in their native form, into flour, giving humans an inexhaustible supply of carbohydrate calories. Domesticating animals and crops gave us an ample supply of food but limited its breadth as we began to rely on only a few sources of nutrition relative to the bounty of foods in the hunter-gatherer diet.

The addition of salt to our food during the Agricultural Era allowed us to extend our food supply year-round without refrigeration. With these advances, man was finally able to put his mind to something other than the daily hunt.

To the lament of every couch potato on Earth, we did not choose to laze around all day with our newfound leisure time. Man put his creative energies into industry and commerce, and a few thousand years later ushered in the Industrial Revolution.

The Industrial Revolution brought even more dramatic changes to our environment. We began to genetically engineer our crops to increase their yield. We invented new animal feeds capable of greatly reducing the time from birth to slaughter. Our plants and animals are no longer plucked from our surroundings but have become our own creations. We created highly processed foods of increasing complexity and added chemicals invented in laboratories to improve taste, texture, and shelf life. In short, we have applied millions of years of evolutionary intelligence to changing our food supply to meet our needs. But what needs were we meeting? Were we trying to make our diets ever healthier or use our intellect to extend our useful lives? Sadly, no. For the sake of this discussion we can summarize our dietary innovations as serving one of three purposes:

1) Palatability. We developed foods that were tasty. Catering to our taste for fatty, salty, or sweet foods, we created foods that satisfied those cravings. We stripped away the fiber, protein, and nutrients to push our happiness buttons with foods that were sweet and savory. We've become so used to spoiling our taste buds that the mere thought of having food that is neither sweet nor savory is instantly rejected by many people (I've seen their faces in my office).

2) Convenience. To satisfy our increasingly busy lives we developed foods that were increasingly convenient. From the invention of sandwiches in the 1800s to microwavable TV dinners and drive-through fast-food restaurants, we made food easier to prepare and faster to eat. The more we advanced as a race, the busier we became, and the less time we had for food preparation.

Thankfully we no longer must hunt our food, but now even the most basic food preparation often seems to be a chore.

3) Ubiquity. Gone are the days of scarcity and famine. Now food is ubiquitous and plentiful, with super-sized portions, all-you-can-eat buffets, and a grocery store or restaurant on every corner. Our genetic engineering, animal husbandry, and advanced agriculture have given us an endless array of inexpensive, readily available foods.

No doubt these alterations to our food supply are not entirely bad—why not have tasty, plentiful, convenient food? The problem is that our bodies simply have not had time to catch up to this new diet. We can innovate and change our food supply exponentially faster than our bodies can evolve. Most of the changes to our food supply have come within the past few hundred years, while evolution is measured in *millions* of years.

YOU'RE NOT SICK, YOU'RE EVOLVING

Our diet today is vastly different from that of our hunter-gatherer ancestors. Today grains and dairy now make up about one-third of the modern diet, yet were unknown only 300 generations ago. A full 70% or more of the calories in a typical, modern day come from foods that simply didn't exist even a few thousand years ago, many of which were added in only the past few decades. In addition to grains and dairy we have added sugars, vegetable oils, salt, and alcohol. It has literally only been five generations since Coca-Cola was first found on market shelves. In evolutionary terms we are in a vastly different environment from that to which we had adapted over millions of years.

Let's put this in the context of natural selection and human evolution. The Agricultural Era (10,000 years ago), and more recently the Industrial Era (200 years ago), ushered in a permanent shift in our environment from a hunter-gatherer diet that was relatively stable for millions of years to a diet consisting largely of foods that were previously unknown.

So what happens when we change our environment? The same thing that happens when every species is faced with a dramatic environmental shift: the fittest survive. A lucky few of us will be genetically able to handle a diet of pizza, Coke, and pasta all day. Everyone has a story of their great grandpa or someone who smoked a pack a day, ate cheeseburgers, and drank whisky yet lived to be ninety-nine years old without ever seeing a doctor. (Not exactly the "fittest" but you get the idea.) On the other end of the bell curve is the poor guy who can't even smell a donut without gaining two pounds.

Most of us are neither morbidly obese nor blessed to be in perfect shape on a diet of Twinkies and Ding Dongs. Instead, most of us see evidence of our poor adaptation to a Western diet in the form of chronic disease. As we age and our bodies fail to adapt to our new habitat, our systems break down. Cholesterol, blood pressure, and blood sugars rise. Arteries become stiff and prone to clogging. Our kidneys fail, our memory fades, and our skin becomes frail and wrinkled. Bones become brittle and break easily. Our balance starts to falter, making those fractures ever more likely. And by the time we are in our seventies, most of us will be on a first name basis with our doctors and know the phone number to the local pharmacy by heart.

This is not to say that modern foods are inherently bad for us—one plate of pasta is not likely to make you ill. However, for most of us, even those of us who eat healthy, these foods have become staples, comprising the *majority* of our diets. As we will see, a lifetime of consuming our current staples - dairy, cereal grains, sugars, salt, and vegetable oils - wreaks havoc with our bodies. Your body will try desperately to adapt to these new foods, but over time, your systems break down and chronic disease and aging are the result. We simply have not evolved to be able to survive on a Western diet *and we won't in this lifetime.*

LET'S GO HOME

The solution to chronic disease and aging is right in front of us: we simply need to return to our natural habitat. Once we start to exercise and eat like our ancestors did, many of these problems will start to go away. We will then need fewer medications, we will have more energy, and our bodies and minds will be sharper. This doesn't mean we need to forgo all our worldly possessions and scour Torrey Pines State Park for food. We have it much better than cavemen ever did—we have the luxury of hunting and gathering our food from restaurants and grocery stores, limiting ourselves to the selections available to our prehistoric ancestors. Now we just need to learn how to do it.

Why can't I just eat healthy again?

You might be thinking that this evolution thing sounds good but isn't any different from anything you've heard before. You might even think that you already do eat all natural foods, so you're already doing this. But the reality is that most of us pay lip service to our nutrition and then kid ourselves that we can be healthy just by eating American food in moderation. Eat smaller portions, choose healthier options, and skip the French fries. Unfortunately, this strategy rarely works. You can lose weight by eating less, but you won't prevent disease or get off your medications unless you choose foods in tune with your evolutionary biology.

In fact, understanding evolution helps explain some of our most basic cravings. Our natural habitat, the one that your body still thinks it is in, lacks two things that you'll find pervasive in our current food supply: concentrated calories and salt. The real world doesn't have readily available sources of fat or carbohydrates; few plants have abundant carbohydrates or sugars, and animal fat is especially difficult to come by. In the real world animals are lean, active creatures and rarely store more fat than they need; most wild animals have little body fat relative to their modern domesticated counterparts. Salt is also virtually unknown in the wild. Since calories and sodium are difficult to find, yet necessary for survival, it is only natural that we developed an evolutionary craving for both. Finding a fruit tree or felling a wild animal might mean the difference between life and death. For millions of years our survival depended on it.

Now our modern world has given us the opportunity to create endless supplies of fat, salt, and sugar. We crave these foods for good reason—your body still thinks you just woke up in the jungle and hit the jackpot. If you've ever scarfed through an entire bag of potato chips (guilty!) you know that the drive to eat so voraciously has to come from a place as visceral as survival.

This evolutionary fact is certainly not lost on anyone in the food business. Sodium, fat, and carbs make it into virtually every processed food, even the so-called healthy ones. We all know that junk food and fast food is packed with all three of these treats—that's what makes them junk food. However, "healthy" processed foods are rarely any better. Tell me, how many people would be above putting a little salt or fat into a protein bar to make it sell better? Carefully read the labels of your favorite health food and you are bound to find a bit of sugar, fat, or salt there to make it more appetizing. Companies don't trust you to buy it if they don't put something in it to make it tasty.

With so many food companies preying on your evolutionary urges it is nearly impossible to get healthy eating processed foods that other people tell you are healthy. You can be sure that there is something in there that you don't need, and it will almost certainly be enough to throw you off track from meeting even modest health-related goals.

If you don't think navigating modern healthy choices is difficult, it helps to see the lengths to which companies will go to convince you that they are pushing healthy foods. Beyond tweaking ingredients to fit generally accepted definitions of healthy foods, companies often just change the definition of "healthy" to meet their needs. Focusing on the calories instead of nutritional value is a favorite tactic. For example, *THE ECONOMIST* reports that Nestlé's nutritional profiling system has identified nearly three-fourths of its food products as being an appropriate part of a healthy diet. Among the "healthy" products: a bite-sized Kit Kat bar. Need I say more?

Talk about mixed messaging— according to Nestlé, a Kit Kat bar is part of a healthy, balanced diet.

Marketers make a living turning the fine print into bold messages that entice you to buy food based on its healthy benefits. But who is defining "healthy"? Don't allow the food companies to define "healthy" for you. My definition is simple, and I encourage you to use it for yourself when evaluating food choices:

"Healthy" means living a long time, free of disease, on as few medications as possible.

If the food in front of you is healthy, it will move you one step closer to adding another day to your life, curing or preventing disease, or getting you off medication. If food doesn't do that, it just isn't healthy.

The ancestral diet—and perhaps only the ancestral diet—lives up to this high standard. You'll see as you go through the following chapters that the ancestral diet is consistent with everything you'll read about good health. It explains why there's so much backlash against grains, why vegetarians get less heart disease, why Atkins helps you lose weight, why Asians live longer, and why Mediterranean cultures have less heart disease. Pretty much anything you've heard about diet is based on our ancestral diet; it's the one thread that ties together everything we know about modern nutrition. It's as though science was not discovering anything new but simply shedding light on what has been there all along.

John E., age 73

When I first started with Dr. Dave I was on a total of six medications, including four for my blood pressure alone. I'd been thinking about diet and exercise for a long time but struggled to put my thoughts into action.

At the same time I was getting more concerned about the side effects of the medications I was taking. My ankles swelled some days. I'd be rushing to the bathroom frequently, and one of the medications warned that it could cause male breast enlargement. I wanted to get off as many medications as possible without compromising my health.

Dr. Dave's exercise and diet program turned out to be the answer. After only a few weeks on the program my blood pressure had come down from the 140/90 range to the 100/70 range. One by one, Dr. Dave and my cardiologist started cutting down my blood pressure medications, and after only a few months I was down to just one. *I dropped three out of four blood pressure medications.* I felt I was on the road to redemption.

One of the most important outcomes of this program was one I didn't see coming. I had an echocardiogram, which showed that years of high blood pressure had taken their toll. Part of my heart muscle had thickened to the point that the blood was no longer flowing effectively with each heartbeat. My cardiologist wanted me to avoid vigorous exercise, so Dr. Dave suggested modifications to the program that enabled me to stay within safe limits while continuing to work toward better health. Since then I've rarely missed a workout and have continued to feel healthier and fitter.

I don't know if I'd ever have made it into the gym or improved my diet if I hadn't met Dr. Dave. His program is truly a blessing.

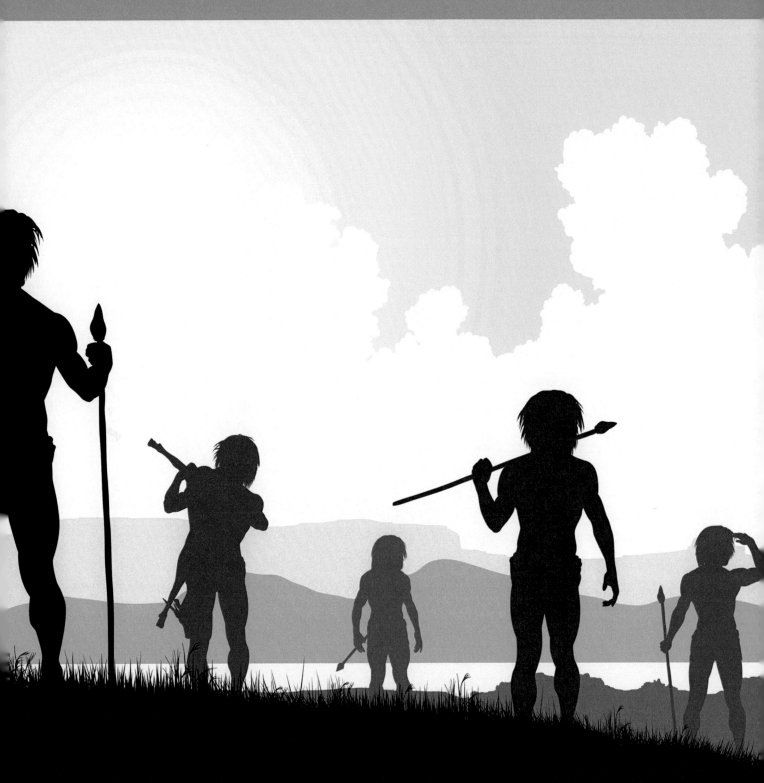

OUR ANCESTRAL DIET

SO WHAT EXACTLY DID OUR DIET LOOK LIKE BEFORE WE STARTED ALTERING IT? Before the advent of modern agriculture you could eat only what you could hunt or gather. Therefore, to get your arms around this concept and apply it in your life you simply need to use your common sense:

If it wasn't around one million years ago, don't eat it.

This one rule will get you closer to good health than any other diet plan I've ever seen, and it doesn't require getting a PhD in clinical nutrition or staying glued to the TV for the latest health tips. Just see if what you are about to put on your plate is new or old, and you'll know what to do. But if you need a quick look at some examples, here they are:

Pre-Agricultural Era Foods: Wild-caught meat and seafood, nuts, fruits, vegetables, eggs, seeds, berries, and water

Modern Industrial Era Foods: Commercially-raised meat and farmed seafood, pasta, bread, rice, dairy, sodas, pastries, sauces, salt, and condiments

The common thread among the pre-Agricultural Era foods is that they were all around one million years ago and none of them need to be altered significantly from their natural form prior to eating. Told you this was going to be easy!

As easy as this is, you'll be better able to stick with this plan if you have a deeper understanding of how our ancestral diet works to help you get and stay healthy. So we're going to keep it as simple as we can, but also take the time to learn about grains, dairy, meats, and other food groups so that you understand the impact each has on your health. By the time you're done with this section, you should have an excellent understanding of how to make your ancestral hunter-gatherer diet work for you.

MEAT ME AT THE CORONARY CARE UNIT

Meat is one of those polarizing topics that gets everyone riled up. If I even suggest giving up red meat entirely, most of my patients just tell me to renew their prescription for Lipitor and forget the diet. The thought of going without burgers and steaks conjures up visions of a lifetime of salads and the conversation is over before it began.

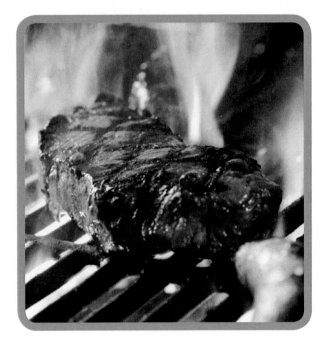

Many years ago Atkins popularized a diet that gave us the perception that perhaps beef and pork were good for you. Intuitively, many of us were skeptical despite our enthusiastic desire to believe this. Wouldn't you love to live on bacon and hamburgers and clear out your arteries at the same time? Unfortunately, we've also all heard that red meat increases the risk of heart attack and stroke. In fact, bookshelves suggest that the vegetarians are winning out in the popularity contest lately, with books like *The China Study* and *Forks Over Knives* promoting a purely vegetarian or vegan diet. So is Atkins right and we should reach for the bacon, or should we all put down our knives and go vegetarian?

Here's where thinking like a caveman sheds some light on the puzzle: looking back to our ancestral roots gives us an answer somewhere in the middle. Historical clues suggest that our ancestors were definitely hunters—the remains of hunting gear and animal carcasses are evidence that meat-eating played a role in our evolution. Researchers speculate that during the caveman days meat probably comprised between one-third and one-half of the calories in our diet, with the remainder of our calories coming from plant sources.

Today we're obviously a far cry from sharpening spears and chasing buffalo. One major difference between us and our ancestors is that our ancestors couldn't stroll down to the local grocery store and pick out a nice rib-eye steak any day of the week. We can guess that meat wasn't on the menu every day simply because hunting wild game is easier said than done (you don't have to outrun a vegetable). Secondly, the animals our ancestors hunted were vastly different from the ones that end up on grocery shelves today. Wild animals, whether bison, elk, or lamb, run around all day, eating nice green, leafy vegetables. They are lean, muscular animals with very little body fat. Even the fat that they do have is a healthier version than what we find in today's store-bought meats. Looking at the way meat is produced today gives us a sense of how different our meat is from that on which we evolved.

Up through the 1940s almost all the beef produced in the U.S. was the product of cows raised on pasture. Unfortunately, raising cows on pasture turns out to be a relatively inefficient way to produce beef. Cows need a lot of grazing area to feed, and during winter or off-season months, the grass is thin and opportunities to graze are limited. If you are in the business of raising and selling cattle, this is a problem in need of a solution. Who wants to wait all winter for a cow to start getting fat again?

The solution to lean cows turned out to be corn and other grains. Starting in the 1950s, commercial farms began to introduce high-energy grain feeds as a way to accelerate the time needed for a calf to reach its slaughter weight. Over the ensuing sixty-odd years, corn-fed beef has become the norm in the United States. Common feeds in addition to good ol' Midwestern corn include barley concentrate, soybean meal, and distillers' grains (corn or wheat byproducts from alcohol fermentation). Other common feeds include animal byproducts (what's left over after all the meat is gone) and waste products (yes, that's right, cow poop). One of the reasons mad-cow disease spread so quickly among cattle is that one sick cow got fed to the others. Makes you pause before reaching for that rib-eye on sale for $4.99 a pound, doesn't it?

Changing the way we feed animals works great for the mass-production of meat products. Compared to their pasture-raised brethren, cows that are raised indoors on a diet of concentrated grains have a shorter time to market (12–18 months vs. 23 months) and generally weigh more at slaughter (around 750 pounds vs. 600 pounds). Basically, you can get 25% more cow in half the time if you forget the grass and feed them everything but the kitchen sink. Definitely good for industry but not so good for your health.

Changing the way we feed our animals has dramatic implications for the nutritional content of the meat we eat. Compared to grain-fed beef, grass-fed beef is leaner, less atherogenic (less likely to block arteries), and has more omega-3s, more vitamins, and more cancer-fighting antioxidants. Let's look at these distinctions in detail:

Leaner: Pastured cows are able to walk around all day, and that exercise means that they are generally leaner than grain-fed cows who sit in a barn all day. In a comparison of grass-fed and grain-fed strip steaks from around the country, the grass-fed steaks were on average 36% leaner.

Less atherogenic: Beef contains saturated fat and cholesterol, both of which will increase your LDL or "bad" cholesterol, contributing to a higher risk of heart attack and stroke. Grass-fed beef has just as much saturated fat and cholesterol as grain-fed beef, but the *type* of saturated fat it has might not raise your cholesterol in the same way. There are several types of saturated fat, some of which are more likely to raise cholesterol and some of which are less likely. Grass-fed beef has about 20% more *stearic acid*, which is a type of saturated fat that does not raise cholesterol. Therefore, the fat content of grass-fed beef is less likely to translate to higher cholesterol levels. Interestingly, stearic acid is also found in chocolate, which may account for some of its health benefits. More on this in a later chapter.

Saturated fat in grass-fed beef is high in the proportion that does not raise LDL or "bad" cholesterol.

More Omega-3: Omega-3 fats are heart-healthy fats that reduce inflammation in the body, improve brain function, and reduce the risk of heart attack and stroke. Omega-6 fats do exactly the opposite, causing inflammation and increasing the risk of disease. We're going to cover this in more detail in the next chapter, but for now, suffice it to say that we want to get more omega-3 and less omega-6. Grass is rich in omega-3, which is then found in the meat we get from pastured cows. In contrast, grains, corn, and soybeans are high in omega-6, which ends up in the meat from grain-fed cows.

The modern diet is heavily skewed toward grains and grain-fed meats, making our diet much higher in inflammatory fats than we want. Our distant ancestors probably had about a 2:1 ratio of omega-6 to omega-3 fat, a level that gives a good balance of inflammation in the body. Today the ratio is closer to 10:1 in favor of pro-inflammatory omega-6. Grass-fed meats have exactly the 2:1 ratio of omega-6 to omega-3 fat that we are striving for in our diet.

---

*Grass-fed beef has the perfect balance
of omega-3 and omega-6 fats.*

High in antioxidants: Grass-fed beef is superior to grain-fed when it comes to the fat soluble vitamins α-tocopherol (vitamin E) and beta-carotene (vitamin A). Fresh grass has about five times more vitamin A than grain or hay, and is rich in vitamin E. Cows are actually very efficient at storing these vitamins and passing them on to you. Interestingly, the antioxidant properties of vitamin E are associated with an increase in the shelf life of grass-fed beef over the grain-fed variety.

---

*Grass-fed beef has over two times more vitamin E
and four times more vitamin A than grain-fed beef.*

*You can actually see the vitamins in grass-fed meats.
The high concentration of carotenoids gives the fat a yellow or red
hue, which can be compared with the stark white of corn-fed beef.*

So is all this actually worth the extra money? The answer depends on how much you like red meat. Clearly, store-bought meat is going to raise your cholesterol levels, fatten you up, and promote inflammation. If you want to get off or stay off cholesterol medications and reduce your risk of bad things happening, you can either forgo red meat entirely (which is a very reasonable option), or keep it in moderation and shop for the grass-fed/grass-finished variety. Expect to pay anywhere from 20–100% more for your purchase, but remember where the savings at the grocery store are coming from—cheap feed, industrialized beef production from penned-in cows, and a process dedicated to making the fattest cow possible in the least amount of time. Is that a part of the food chain you want to be a part of?

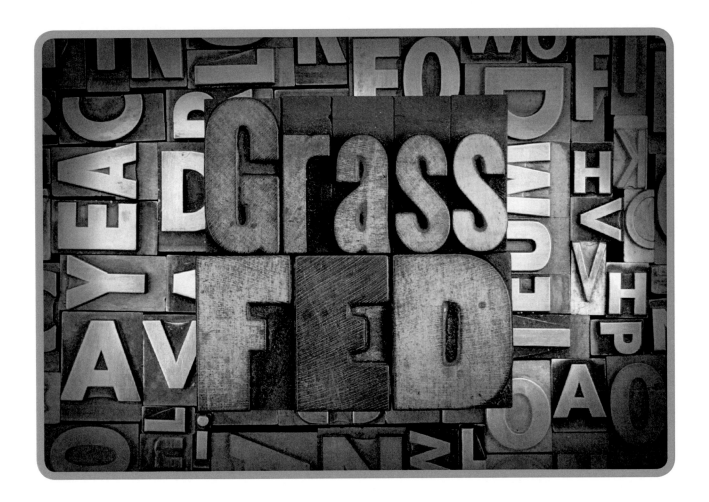

GRASS-FED OR GRASS-FINISHED?

Most cows, even grain-fed ones, are raised on pasture for at least a few months after birth. It is only during the last several months of their lives that they are transferred to feed lots to be fattened up for slaughter. Since it takes only a few months for the fatty acid profile of the diet to be reflected in the meat, it is these last few months that determine the composition of the meat in the store.

Grass-fed meats are generally considered to be grass-fed throughout their lives; however, it is possible that even a "grass-fed" cow might have been finished on grain for a few months prior to slaughter. Grass-finished meat, as the name implies, comes from cows that consume fresh grasses in the months before slaughter. If you can't verify with the producer whether grass-fed is also grass-finished, keep shopping.

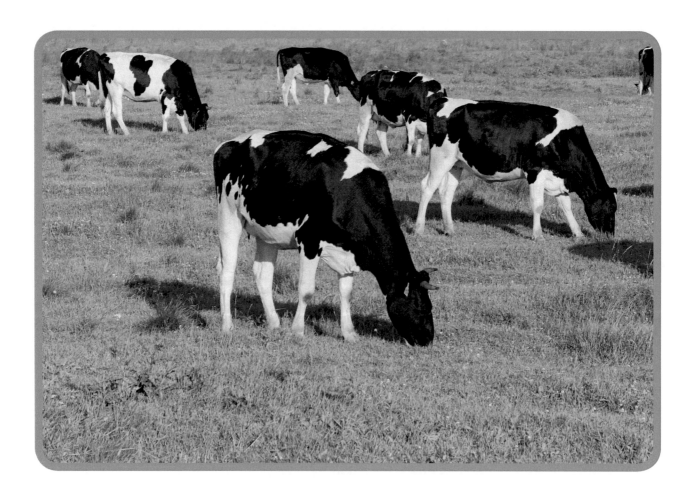

Chew on this...

Thanks to a quirk of cow biology, grass-fed beef is one of the best dietary sources of the cancer-fighting compound conjugated linoleic acid (CLA). A cow does not just chew and digest food like we do—it ruminates on it. Grasses, once chewed, are passed to the rumen, which is the digestive equivalent of a fermentation vat. Bacteria in the rumen ferment the grass, often for days, prior to digestion. During this rumination process, a bacterium called *butyrivibrio fibrisolvens* transforms omega-6 and omega-3 fatty acids in the grass into conjugated linoleic acid. The more grass the cow chews, the higher the amounts of CLA in the meat. All ruminants, including cows, sheep, goats, and deer, have high concentrations of CLA provided they consume a grass diet.

CLA has been shown to have potent cancer-fighting ability. In animal models, CLA inhibits the growth of breast, prostate, and gastrointestinal cancers. A recommended intake has not been established, although estimates range from 95 milligrams to up to 3,000 milligrams daily. About 5% of the fat in grass-fed beef is CLA, so a typical quarter pound serving of 80% lean ground beef has about 1,000 milligrams of CLA, right in the middle of the recommended range.

> ### *Understanding the Labels on Red Meat–Common Pitfalls*
>
> **GRASS-FED BUT CORN-FINISHED** Grass-finished beef has all the health benefits of grass feeding. Make sure that your grass-fed beef was actually finished on grass as well. Corn-finished is corn-fed.
>
> **ORGANIC** Organic meats are all-natural, but corn is as natural as you can get. Avoiding the antibiotics and growth hormones used in breeding cattle may offer some health benefits, but is unlikely to truly move the needle with respect to measurable health outcomes.
>
> **VEGETARIAN DIET** A vegetarian diet certainly includes corn or other grains. Certain feeds may contain the remains of other animals, including animals that were not fit for human consumption or the waste products after slaughter. A vegetarian diet excludes these animal products but is not equivalent to grass-fed.

Before we stock our freezer with an entire grass-fed cow, it's worth mentioning that grass-fed meat is not necessarily the whole story; a few other factors may influence the role of meat in the development of heart disease. Dr. Stanley Hazen at the Cleveland Clinic has shown that two molecules found in high concentrations in meat–l-carnitine and choline–may contribute to the development of heart disease. These compounds are metabolized by intestinal bacteria, which convert them into trimethylamine n-oxide (TMAO). This TMAO is reabsorbed further down the intestines and enters the circulation. TMAO levels in the bloodstream interfere with cholesterol metabolism, preventing good cholesterol from doing its job of removing cholesterol from circulation. Cholesterol is then more likely to build up on the arterial wall, putting you at risk of heart attacks and strokes.

There is also a strong argument to be made that cooking red meat at high temperatures both creates carcinogens and potentially increases the risks of heart disease. A typical grill might generate temperatures of 500 degrees to 1500 degrees or higher at the surface of the meat, creating the characteristic charred surface that seals in the juices. Unfortunately, these high heats may also be oxidizing the fat in the meat, creating free radicals that become a precursor for aging, tissue damage, heart disease, and cancer.

Last but not least, it is worth mentioning that not all meat is the same. So far we've been talking about real meat, right from the source. It should go without saying that you should steer clear of artificial or highly processed meats like salami, sausages, and hot dogs. These meats are packed with fat—way more than any natural meat—plus they have other preservatives such as sodium and nitrites that aren't doing anything to promote your health. Do yourself a favor and limit yourself to meats that your ancestors enjoyed.

So whether it's the choline, carnitine, saturated fat, cholesterol, preservatives, or oxidized lipids in meat that serves as the link to disease, that link definitely exists. If that's all you need to hear to put down your steak knife for good, you'll probably be better off. There's no compelling reason to have red meat in the diet other than taste; however, for many people, cutting out the red meat is a deal-breaker right from the beginning. They're simply not ready to give up their backyard barbeque or the occasional steak for dinner. If you're one of them, you're probably already glazing over at all this red-meat bashing. So what can you do if you want to have your steak and eat it, too?

Let's start with the basics. Stop buying hot dogs, salami, and other processed meats. The cavemen didn't eat them and neither should you. Next up, stick to grass-fed meat, even if it costs you more. You'll get a healthier cut of meat and mitigate some of the risk from eating artificially fattened cows. Besides, you'll be saving money on medications before long. Now we just need to find an acceptable limit for how much red meat we can safely tolerate in our diet.

A landmark heart disease prevention trial published in *The New England Journal of Medicine* in 2013 may give us this answer. The PRIMED trial included well over 7,000 people and looked at how diet affected the risk of heart disease. Most people in the trial were overweight and had one or more risk factors for heart disease, such as high blood pressure or high cholesterol. The investigators found that a Mediterranean diet (more on this later) was associated with a 30% reduction in heart disease over the five years of the trial. What is interesting is that the low risk group didn't avoid red meat altogether, they just limited themselves to less than one serving of red meat per day. Even with eating red meat *almost* every day (but not *every* day) the study participants drastically lowered their risk of heart disease.

What does all this mean? It means that you can get healthy and stay healthy without necessarily taking red meat off the menu. Think about what this PRIMED trial showed: you can eat red meat *almost every day* and still cut your risk of heart disease by a third. As we'll later see, you can also dramatically lower your cholesterol while eating red meat as long as you stick to lean, grass-fed cuts and keep it in moderation. Who would have thought you could get healthy, reduce your medications, and still eat burgers?

It is important to note that there is nothing wrong with a meat-free diet; in fact, eliminating red meat altogether will certainly improve your chances of living a long time free of cardiovascular diseases and cancer. But if you enjoy red meat you need not forgo it altogether. Like our caveman ancestors, you simply must "hunt" for free-range or wild-caught meat and choose the absolute leanest cuts possible. I will warn you that this may cost you a bit more unless you really *are* a hunter, but it allows guilt-free enjoyment of meats without undue health risks. Better your money goes to a local cattle rancher than to Pfizer.

SO WHERE AM I SUPPOSED TO GET MY PROTEIN?

Let's say you've decided to put down your steak knife and pick up a fork. The next question is: where are you going to get your protein? Thankfully, red meat gets most of the bad rap when it comes to disease promotion. Now that we're clear on what to do with our red meat cravings, navigating the rest of the animal kingdom in search of healthy protein sources is easy.

Much of what we learned about beef applies to other animal and seafood products as well. Stick to lean cuts of pork, chicken, lamb, fish, or whatever else you care for. Even better, seek out pasture-raised or wild-caught animal products. You want to lean toward a higher amount of protein and less fat. Pound for pound, protein is more satiating than either fat or carbohydrates. When cooking, go easy on the flame broiling and try not to char the heck out of your food on the grill. Higher cooking temperatures may oxidize fats and sugars in the meat and contribute to the aging process.

It is also worth mentioning that abstaining from meat doesn't mean that you need to panic about finding protein in your diet. There's plenty of protein in plants as well. A handful of nuts or two cups of vegetables each have about 6–10 grams of protein, which is about one-sixth the daily requirement for an average adult. As long as you stick to all-natural foods, you'll get plenty of protein during the day to meet your body's needs.

Here are some examples of healthy, lean cuts of meat and some fattier cuts to be avoided.

Healthy, lean animal products

Beef flank steak, sirloin and top sirloin, lean ground beef (> 90% lean), top round, eye of round, bottom round, and chuck steak
Pork loin or loin chops
Chicken or turkey breast
Egg whites
Game meat
Fish
Most shellfish

Fatty choices to be avoided

Beef rib-eye, ground beef < 90% lean, filet mignon, T-bone, skirt steak, NY strip steak, porterhouse, and flap steak
Pork shoulder or bacon
Chicken and turkey wings, thighs, or legs
Egg yolks

DOES GRASS-FED MATTER FOR OTHER ANIMALS?

It does, but beef tops the list of meats consumed in the U.S. so changing the way we enjoy beef makes a big difference when it comes to measurable health outcomes. According to the AMI (American Meat Institute), over half of household spending on meat goes to red meat (including beef and pork), with just over a third going to poultry and less than 10% spent on fish. That being said, all animal products are better for you if the animals are fed their native diet. Pastured meats may be available at your local specialty grocer and can also be found online at eatwild.com or localharvest.org. Both sites will give you options for finding local farms that raise their livestock on grass and natural foods. If you must get store-bought meat that isn't pastured, keep it lean and keep the portions small. Load up on vegetables instead.

GOING AGAINST THE GRAINS

Wheat, rye, barley, corn, and other cereal grains are another controversial topic in health circles. Once the staple of a healthy diet, grains have come under increasing scrutiny for their role in modern health problems such as the ones we address here.

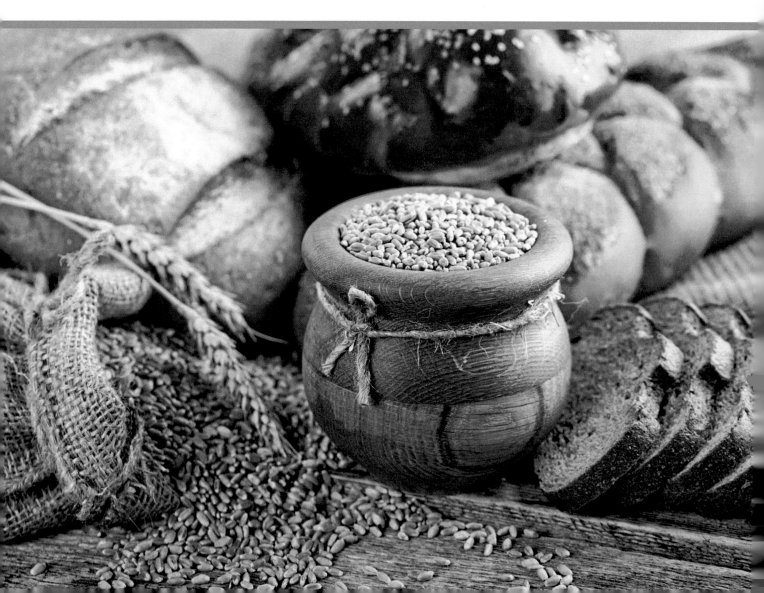

Wheat must be processed to be consumed, and that technology did not exist until roughly 10,000 years ago. If you've ever seen wheat growing in the field, you understand that it is not an obvious food source. Grains must be crushed and the outer hull removed in order to access the digestible innards. Once you grind grains into flour, you still don't have food yet—or at least anything resembling a palatable food worth the effort you've put in so far. Our distant ancestors would probably walk right through an entire field of wheat to find something edible on the other side. What this means is we haven't had time to evolve and adapt to the impact wheat and other grains have on our health.

The first problem posed by the introduction of wheat products into our modern diet is that they are a concentrated source of calories. Especially when processed into pasta or bread, wheat tends to add a great deal of calories to our typical diet (often 20-25% of our daily total). With these calories comes little else of nutritional value. Wheat has relatively few micronutrients or vitamins, especially when compared with vegetables and meat. As a source of fiber, even whole grain products don't really stack up. Whole grain bread provides about 2 grams of fiber per 100 calories. Compare this to broccoli, with 4 grams of fiber for 30 calories. You would need 200 calories of bread to get the same fiber as 30 calories of broccoli!

WHOLE GRAIN, WHOLE CARB

The problems with grains are compounded by the fact that they make up such a large proportion of our total food intake. Think about a typical "healthy" day. You might start with whole grain cereal or a muffin for breakfast, a nice chicken sandwich on whole wheat bread for lunch, and maybe even brown rice with meat and vegetables and some bread with dinner. By the end of the day you may have had as many as 4-5 servings of grains, maybe more. Remember, cavemen had zero.

Unless you are burning serious calories, all that carbohydrate is just confusing your body. Remember that your body still thinks that you are back in the jungle where there's practically no carbohydrates. Citrus fruits and root vegetables are the few exceptions to the rule that the wild is essentially a low-carb environment.

Now, let's say all of a sudden (in evolutionary terms) you scarf down a plate of pasta and dump 400 calories of carbohydrates into your small intestine. For argument's sake, let's also assume that you're not about to outrun a lion or train for the Boston marathon. Your plate of pasta goes right to the liver where it must be either stored or burned for energy. This process of metabolizing carbohydrates is driven by the hormone **insulin**. The carbohydrate rush triggers your pancreas to secrete insulin, which then tells the liver to start turning that carbohydrate into fat. Your liver breaks down the sugars in pasta into individual subunits that can be reassembled into fatty acids. The fatty acids produced from sugar are combined into **triglycerides**, which are the body's standard storage form of fat. These triglycerides are then sent off to your adipose tissue for storage. Now, if this happens once or twice, your body can handle it. Your insulin levels shoot up, sugar turns into fat, and the triglycerides are stored for the next fast when you'll need the calories.

But what if the carbs keep coming or the fast never happens? Your body did not evolve to accommodate persistently high insulin levels, and your pancreas wasn't meant to churn out massive amounts of insulin to accommodate a lifetime of carb intake.

Here's what happens if we keep this up for a few decades. First, you'll notice that you are starting to store fat around your midsection. This fat packs in and around the abdominal organs, just where you need it the least. The fat begins to interfere with normal organ function, primarily in the liver. This is important since the liver is the first stop for food after it is digested and absorbed.

Around the same time, your triglyceride levels in the blood start to rise as your body has trouble finding a home for all of the processed carbohydrate. Your fat cells stop dividing sometime in your childhood, meaning that you have a fixed amount of fat cells as an adult in which to store excess calories. As these fat cells start to fill up, triglycerides and fatty acids start ending up in the blood stream instead of being safely stored away for future use.

Your fat cells, now swollen and unable to function properly, start to malfunction in other ways. Fat cells aren't just storage units for excess calories; they are constantly communicating with the rest of your organs to regulate appetite and metabolism. The hormone **adiponectin** is produced by adipocytes (fat cells) and is essential for the normal functioning of insulin and its receptor. Once these fat cells swell up to capacity, adiponectin levels drop. With low levels of this important cytokine, insulin receptors start to malfunction. The receptors no longer bind as well to insulin, so you need more insulin to get the same effect. This means that the pancreas has to start working overtime, cranking out ever-increasing amounts of insulin to get the same job done. Over the years this cycle perpetuates itself as more carbs lead to ever-increasing levels of triglycerides and worse functioning of the insulin receptors.

Leptin is another hormone secreted by adipocytes as well as by your gut tissues. Leptin is the hormonal link between your stomach, fat cells, and your appetite. When you have a big meal, leptin is released from your intestinal tract to tell your brain to stop eating. Also, when your fat cells start to fill up (i.e., when you gain weight) your leptin levels rise, telling your brain to decrease your appetite. As you might guess, your ancestors didn't have perpetually high leptin levels simply because they didn't have the luxury of carrying around an extra twenty pounds year after year. Any excess weight they had was likely to be put to work keeping them alive all winter.

In prehistoric times as well as today, leptin was an important signal to help keep your appetite in check. But that extra weight around your midsection may be screwing up the transmission. Ever tune someone out when they're nagging you incessantly? Your brain does the same thing. All those fat cells keep cranking out leptin and eventually your brain just stops listening. Once your brain becomes resistant to leptin, there's no feedback in place to stop the appetite, and all you're left with is that evolutionary urge to keep eating until you simply can't have another bite. Of course, this leads to more fat and more leptin resistance in a vicious cycle.

So now your "healthy" whole grain diet is slowly causing your triglycerides to creep up, your adiponectin levels to drop, and your leptin levels to rise. This usually is associated with an increase in the diameter of your midsection (still fit into your college wardrobe?) and signals the first steps toward diabetes. In fact there is good evidence that a high triglyceride level is an early warning sign of impending diabetes.

About one in three adults has high triglycerides and two out of three are overweight. This means that most people are somewhere on the track to getting diabetes—the only question is; when are you going to get off the track?

LOW FAT, BUT NOT THE GOOD KIND

While grains are admittedly low-fat, the fat they do have is predominantly in the form of omega-6 fatty acids. As we will later see, these fats are highly pro-inflammatory and have been linked to worse cardiovascular outcomes (i.e., greater risk of dying from heart disease). As we shift our diet away from cereal grains, our bodies become less prone to inflammation, reducing our risk of heart disease as well as other inflammatory diseases such as asthma or arthritis.

DON'T BE A GLUTEN

So if the carbs in wheat aren't healthy and the fat isn't healthy then at least wheat protein must be healthy, right? Sorry, but no. Wheat protein, otherwise known as gluten, may be the worst offender in the entire crop. Gluten is relatively new to our evolutionary diet; it wasn't until about 10,000 years ago that man was first exposed to this protein. Consequently, our digestive tract and the rest of our body haven't yet had time to figure out what to do with it.

Many of us have some degree of intolerance to wheat protein. In its worst manifestations, usually associated with a true allergy and detectable blood levels of antibodies to gluten, gluten sensitivity can contribute to anemia, bone loss (osteoporosis), erosions of tooth enamel, and stunted growth. Other symptoms associated with gluten intolerance include abdominal pain, rash, headache, fatigue, "foggy mind," diarrhea and depression. Just one look at this list of symptoms and it's easy to see that many of us might be suffering from low levels of gluten sensitivity. Gluten sensitivity ranks right up there with raising children and sitting through staff meetings among the top causes of headaches, fatigue and "foggy mind."

So how do you know if you've got gluten sensitivity? In severe cases, gluten allergy, otherwise known as celiac disease, can be diagnosed by checking the blood for antibodies to gluten. Your doctor can check for these antibodies on a routine blood test; however, only a small minority of patients with gluten intolerance will actually have measurable levels of antibodies in their bloodstream. For most people the only way to diagnose gluten intolerance is to stop eating wheat products and see if they start feeling better. It usually takes at least 2 weeks or more to see a difference, but it is likely worth the wait.

In summary, wheat is a relatively new addition to the human diet, has minimal nutritional value, is a source of excess calories, promotes inflammation, and has the potential to disrupt normal digestion and leave you feeling tired and lousy. It's a long-winded way of saying what you probably already know – bagels just aren't good for you. Now let's turn our attention to a few other grains that we are going to be avoiding and learn why.

EAT YOUR CORN LIKE A CAVEMAN

Among the cereal grains, corn has the highest fat content, which is one of the reasons that corn oil has become a popular commercial oil. That, plus generous taxpayer subsidies, means that corn oil finds its way into most processed foods. Corn oil is found in most undifferentiated vegetable oils and turns up frequently in restaurants as well.

Corn oil is predominantly omega-6, like other grains, only corn has more of it. Also like other grains, corn contains plenty of carbs and nothing of nutritional value that cannot be had elsewhere. I would suggest avoiding corn in your diet, especially if it is milled into a carbohydrate-laden delicacy like a tortilla or enchilada. If you want to enjoy corn, do it the way our ancestors did and chew it right off the cob.

RICE, IT'S JUST ANOTHER GRAIN

As with wheat, rice must be processed to be eaten. The outer husk must be cracked and removed before the brown rice is revealed underneath. This can be done with a mortar and pestle or by modern machinery. Before the Agricultural Era, it is doubt-ful that anyone put in the effort to make rice part of the diet. You can just picture some caveman banging away with two rocks pulling the husks off one grain of rice at a time. He'd probably die of starvation before getting a bowl together.

It was only about 10,000 years ago that Asian cultures introduced rice as a staple food. Now rice is second only to corn in global agricultural production and takes its place as another high-carb, low-nutrient staple of our diet. Even brown rice, long considered a healthy food, is high in calories and carbohydrates relative to its nutritional content.

QUINOA, NO EXCEPTION TO THE RULE

Quinoa is technically a seed but has a nutritional composition similar to that of grains. While there is certainly a case to be made favoring quinoa over grains, it is not strong enough to merit bending the rules of the ancestral diet. Quinoa was not part of the human diet until a few thousand years ago when it was first cultivated in South America. Quinoa's appeal as a high-protein grain substitute starts to diminish when it is compared to grains and to the whole foods that constituted our evolutionary diet—lean meats, nuts, fruits, and vegetables. Vegetables have more fiber and vitamins, while meats have more protein.

Nutrition information for one cup, cooked

	QUINOA	BROWN RICE	SWEET POTATOES	BROCCOLI	GREEN BEANS
Calories	222	216	180	55	44
Protein (g)	8.1	5.0	4.0	3.7	2.4
Fat (g)	3.6	1.8	0.3	0.6	0.4
Fiber (g)	5.2	3.5	6.6	5.1	4.0
Carbohydrate (g)	39.4	44.8	41.4	11.2	9.9

As the above table shows, even "healthy" grains and quinoa have a lot of calories, carbohydrates, and fat compared to vegetables. Starchy tubers such as sweet potatoes, still high in carbohydrates and calories, are lower in fat and higher in fiber than grains. Clearly, cup for cup green vegetables are superior sources of fiber and even protein. In fact, two cups of broccoli would provide half the calories, twice the fiber, nearly the same amount of protein, and one-third the fat of one cup of quinoa. Tell me that doesn't make you consider a second serving of broccoli over that "healthy" quinoa.

MILK IS FOR BABIES

Dairy products are definitely a new addition to our human diet. Even if you were to catch up to a cow in the wild, there's little possibility that she would just sit there while you tried to milk her. Humans are supposed to just have human breast milk, and when that's over there's no more dairy. We generally lose the ability to process lactose, the primary sugar in milk products, after childhood. In fact, only about half of adults possess the lactase enzyme needed to digest dairy. This should serve as a reminder that evolution is slow to catch up to dietary changes.

So what's wrong with dairy? First of all, it wasn't part of our hunter-gather evolutionary diet, so as with wheat, ingesting dairy is playing Russian roulette with your genetics.

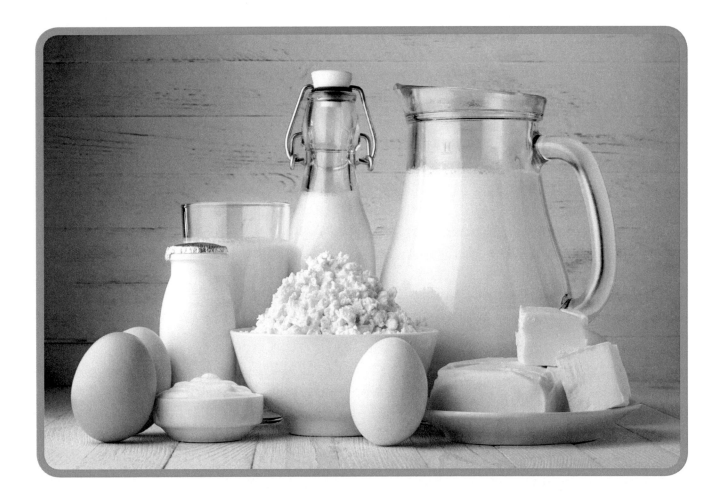

Let's look at what actually makes up most dairy products. Milk, even fat-free milk, is a concentrated source of calories and sugars that are rapidly absorbed. Our bodies simply aren't used to such quantities of sugar (from any source) on a regular basis. That's why skim milk is a less than ideal "healthy" option, especially if you are diabetic or heading that way. For that matter, drinking any calories from juice, milk, or sweetened beverages is generally a bad idea.

The fat in dairy products, such as butter, cheese, cream, and milk, is predominantly saturated fat and pro-inflammatory omega-6. Cheese is one of the most consumed dairy products in the American diet. From the morning omelet to the afternoon sandwich and pizza for dinner, cheese shows up pretty regularly on the menu. This is unfortunate since cheese happens to be packed with sodium and fat, setting you up for the high blood pressure and high cholesterol that keeps Pfizer and our cardiac cath lab in business. No cheese, no trip to the cath lab.

WHAT ABOUT MY CALCIUM AND VITAMIN D?

While there are benefits associated with nonfat dairy products, such as calcium and vitamin D (in fortified products), these can be obtained elsewhere without the excess sugar calories in milk. Vitamin D is super-important, not only for healthy bones, but also for preventing cancer and diabetes, among other things. Despite its importance, vitamin D is not normally found in our food supply unless we put it there; only a few foods like salmon and cod liver oil have appreciable amounts of this vitamin. Humans rely on sun exposure for our bodies to produce the active form of vitamin D; however, even in San Diego, few of us get enough sun exposure to reach adequate vitamin D levels. Skip ahead to the end to read more about vitamin D, but for now I'll just say that taking a supplement of 1,000–2,000 units (U) daily is a good idea for all but the most devout sunbathers.

Calcium is a basic building block of bone but is also important for cellular functioning throughout the body. For example, the flow of calcium across cell membranes generates movement in muscles throughout the body, including the heart. Obviously, keeping the heart beating is more important than bone strength in the short run, so your body tends to treat bones as an inventory of stored calcium. If there isn't enough calcium in the diet, we start to pull calcium from bones, reducing their strength.

Doctors generally recommend getting 1,200 mg of calcium and about 400 mg of magnesium daily to prevent bone losses. These numbers are still controversial, since the data is not conclusive as to how much calcium is the right amount. In fact, while calcium supplementation has been associated with a decreased risk of fractures in the elderly, there is also mounting evidence that calcium supplementation may lead to an increased risk of heart attacks. Interestingly, a high-calcium diet is apparently not associated with any increased cardiac risk.

So it is too early to say that taking calcium supplements is necessary, but certainly there is an argument to be made for including calcium-rich foods in the diet. Luckily for us, there's plenty of calcium and magnesium in natural foods beyond dairy. Soybeans and dark green vegetables have an abundance of calcium. Nuts and seeds are also rich sources of calcium. Most other natural foods have around 40–80 milligrams per serving. Over the course of the day, a balanced diet of meats, fish, nuts, and vegetables will provide plenty of calcium—easily enough to keep your bones strong and healthy.

	SERVING SIZE	CALCIUM (mg)	MAGNESIUM (mg)
Soybeans	1 cup boiled	261	108
Turnip greens	1 cup cooked	249	32
Spinach	1 cup cooked	245	157
Almonds	2 oz. (about 44 nuts)	152	158
Broccoli	2 cups cooked	122	48
Kale	1 cup raw	100	31
Arugula	3 cups raw	96	28
Sesame seeds	1 tbsp.	88	32
Figs	3 large figs	67	33
Orange	1 medium fruit	60	15
Walnuts	½ cup chopped	57	92

But I thought Greek yogurt was healthy!

Greek yogurt is a popular dairy item and is frequently perceived to be a healthy food. Yes, Greek yogurt is high in protein and calcium, and can be fat-free, or nearly so. So far so good; however, Greek yogurt still has lactose in it, which most of us can't digest properly. Furthermore, most of us enjoy Greek yogurt with one or more yummy flavors, like honey or strawberry. Those flavors can be a big problem—next time you pick up your favorite brand of Greek yogurt read how much sugar is in those fruity flavors. If you must include plain, nonfat Greek yogurt in your diet, I won't argue, but stay away from the flavored kinds. When in doubt, I'd say don't bend the rules and stay true to your natural diet.

AN EGG A DAY KEEPS THE DOCTOR AWAY

The question of whether or not eggs are healthy is often more perplexing than the question of which came first between the chicken and the egg. Despite their bad rap, studies have largely vindicated the egg of its early characterization as an unhealthy food that caused heart disease. As with meat, looking at this chicken-egg problem through the eyes of our ancestors gives us an answer that makes sense and is consistent with medical research.

Eggs are available in the wild and were certainly part of the ancestral diet; however, one million years ago they were a lot harder to come by than they are today. To enjoy the prehistoric egg breakfast our ancestors had to find a bird's nest and pray that there were eggs in there. Even if they were lucky enough to accomplish this, they'd be unlikely to get anything as richly rewarding as the Grade A Extra Large eggs we find at the local supermarket. Wild bird eggs on average would be much smaller than their modern cultivated equivalents. So, while eggs were part of the hunter-gatherer diet, they were hardly a staple before agriculture made them plentiful.

Today we should think about eggs in these evolutionary terms: they are a healthy addition to our diet but should be enjoyed in moderation. Studies show that an average of one whole egg per day does not increase the risk of heart disease and actually may reduce your risk of stroke. Although eggs are rich in cholesterol, moderate egg intake is unlikely to raise your cholesterol significantly.

I would suggest enjoying no more than one whole egg per day and as many egg whites as you like; for example, you could start your day with a scramble of one whole egg and up to 3 additional egg whites. When at the grocery store, look for eggs that are enriched in omega-3—the extra expense is worth it. Read ahead to the section on healthy fats to learn more about the role of omega-3 in the diet.

An average of one egg a day is good for your health.
Egg whites can be enjoyed without limitation.
Always opt for eggs enriched with omega-3 when available.

EAT YOUR VEGGIES, BUT KEEP YOUR EYE ON THE GI

Vegetables, green ones in particular, are to be enjoyed to your heart's content (literally). Green vegetables have a plethora of vitamins and minerals but supply very few carbohydrates. For this reason alone, green vegetables should be a dietary staple for everyone, especially those with diabetes, high blood sugar, or high triglycerides. Making green, leafy vegetables a true staple of the diet takes a little work since many of us think of veggies as salad fixings and nothing else. In fact, most people don't eat a full serving of vegetables until the evening meal, missing out on a whole day's worth of veggies.

In order to really increase your veggie intake you've got to make a conscious effort to start including them literally from the time you get out of bed. Veggies for breakfast, lunch, and dinner, every day. Don't panic—when we get to the recipes you'll see how easy it can be. I have been pleasantly surprised that most people actually enjoy having veggies this often once they learn some good recipes.

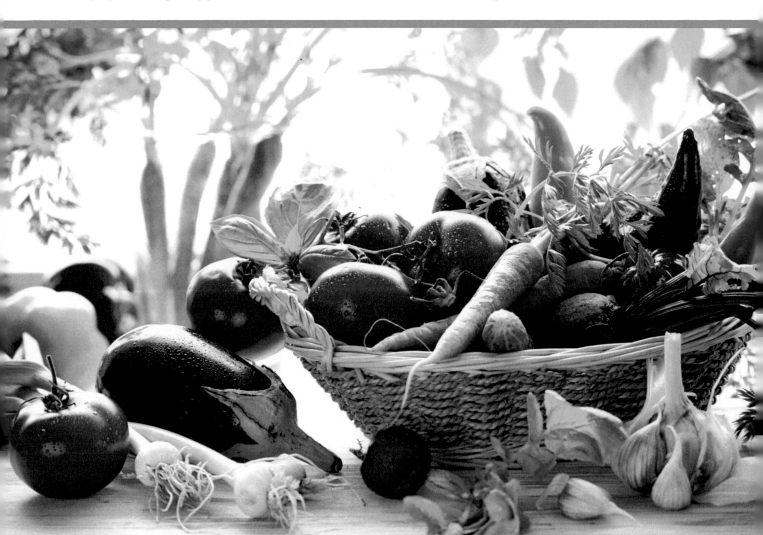

When venturing away from green veggies into colored varieties we have the opportunity to load up on more vitamins like A and C, but also run the risk of loading up on unwanted sugars from starchy tubers. Most of us will be able to tell which veggies are starchy and which are not (clearly, a red pepper and a sweet potato have vastly different calorie counts); however, to eliminate any doubt it helps to introduce a tiny bit of calculation into our discussion.

Most people with diabetes are familiar with the concept of the glycemic index (here's the GI). For the rest of us, the glycemic index is a way to measure how much your blood sugar levels rise after eating one gram of carbohydrate of a certain food. A score of 100 is equivalent to that of pure glucose, and lower numbers are essentially better numbers. A glycemic index of 0 implies that your blood sugars would not rise at all after eating.

The glycemic index therefore gives us a great way to look at starchy vegetables and how they should factor into our diet. In addition to steering clear of processed foods, we want to steer clear of natural foods that are going to affect our body in similar, harmful ways. One such way is by raising our blood sugars and hindering our efforts to lose weight, stay trim, and avoid diabetes.

Take a look at the following table. Foods that are high in fiber and low in sugar are at the bottom of the table, with starchy foods being higher up. Potatoes, which have plenty of starch and little fiber, rank at the very top with a glycemic index nearly equal to that of pure sugar.

On the lower half of the table are the foods we want to emphasize in the diet: most legumes, fruits, and low-glycemic tubers, such as carrots and sweet potatoes. Peanuts have a very low-glycemic index of nearly zero. Remember that the GI only applies to carbs—*any foods with zero carbs, such as nuts, meat, fish, eggs, and green vegetables have a glycemic index of zero.* This means that these foods can be enjoyed with complete abandon without worrying about raising your blood sugars.

Also, note where gluten-free pasta lands on the chart—way at the top. This is why going gluten-free might be the answer to celiac disease or gluten sensitivity but won't get you all the way to good health. Keeping processed foods in the diet means continuing to challenge your ability to regulate blood sugars, leading eventually to diabetes and other metabolic problems.

GLYCEMIC INDEX OF SELECTED FOODS

	GLYCEMIC INDEX
Potato (baked, w/o skin)	98
Gluten-free pasta	78
Cornflakes cereal	74
Potato (baked, w/ skin)	69
Pineapple (raw)	66
Beetroot	64
Brown rice	62
Pasta	61
Yam (peeled, boiled)	54
Pumpkin (boiled)	51
Corn (on the cob)	48
Banana (raw)	47
Sweet potato (boiled, w/o skin)	46
Sweet potato (boiled, w/ skin)	44
Apple (raw)	40
Apricot (raw)	34
Black eyed peas (boiled)	33
Chickpeas (boiled)	33
Pear (raw)	33
Oranges (raw)	33
Carrots (peeled, boiled)	33
Butter beans (boiled)	26
Soybeans (boiled)	20
Kidney beans (boiled)	19
Peanuts	7

Anyone with diabetes should enjoy foods with a moderate glycemic index sparingly, if at all.

*Avoid even natural foods like brown rice
and potatoes that have a high glycemic index.*

*A low-glycemic index diet has been associated with
weight loss, lower blood sugar and cholesterol levels,
and a lower risk of diabetes and heart disease.*

I LOVE FRUITS AND VEGETABLES. I THINK I'LL JUST STICK WITH FRUIT.

Before you go equating fruits and vegetables there's one huge point worth making. Although fruits are more nutritious than processed foods, they aren't quite on the same level as a vegetable. Once upon a time this might have been the case, back when fruits were found wild in their natural form; however, today's store-bought fruits are vastly different from those our ancestors would have enjoyed. They are larger, sweeter, and have less fiber than their wild counterparts. In fact, the sugar composition of many fruits is more similar to that of a cookie than a vegetable.

Let's start with the size and composition of the fruit. Modern fruits are selectively bred to be much larger than their wild counterparts. Most of the fiber in fruits is in the peel and the seeds; even though the peel makes up only a small fraction of the total volume of the fruit, it contains fully half the fiber. Smaller fruits have more seeds and peel relative to the amount of pulp, and consequently contain more fiber than typical store-bought fruit. If you doubt that we've engineered our food this way, just look for seedless grapes or watermelon growing in the wild.

The sugar content of fruit has also changed from our ancestral days. Fruits today are selectively bred to be much sweeter than wild fruits. There are three sugars found in fruits: **glucose**, **fructose**, and **sucrose**. Glucose and fructose are simple sugars that are absorbed in our intestines and metabolized into energy. Sucrose, found in table sugar, is a larger molecule made up of one fructose and one glucose bound together. This bond is then broken and the individual sugars are metabolized separately. All three sugars are found in nature.

Of the three sugars, glucose is considered the least sweet by humans. On a scale of sweetness (based on the sweetness of sucrose), glucose ranks lowest at 80, sucrose is the reference of 100, and fructose ranks highest at 140. Foods that have more fructose and sucrose will be perceived to be sweeter than those that have more glucose. Consequently, if you want to make food taste sweeter, you just remove glucose and add sucrose and fructose.

That is pretty much what we've done with fruits over time. Sucrose and fructose make up over 95% of the sugar in a modern fruit yet are less than half of the sugar in wild fruit. With so much sucrose and fructose (table sugar and high-fructose corn syrup) and so little fiber, you can see how a mango may have more in common with a cookie than you thought.

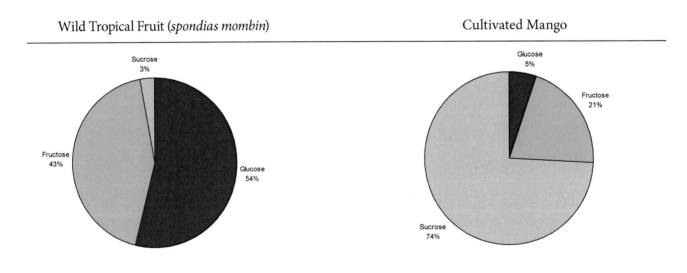

MAN CANNOT LIVE ON LEGUMES ALONE

For those of us who are not botanists, a legume is a plant that has a seed and a pod. Examples include peas, peanuts, beans, soybeans, and lentils, all of which were certainly around long before the age of agriculture. As a food source today, legumes make an excellent addition to the diet. They are generally low in fat, high in protein, and packed with fiber. They also have a low-glycemic index, making them easy on your pancreas and liver.

Legumes occasionally get a bad rap for their "anti-nutrients," which are compounds that may have deleterious effects when ingested. These include the **trypsin inhibitor**, which prevents the body from digesting proteins; **hemagglutinins** or **lectins**, which coagulate blood and may damage intestinal walls during digestion; and **phytates**, which inhibit the absorption of minerals. These anti-nutrients have a toxic effect on the body, making legumes a poor food source in the wild.

Thankfully, there is an easy way to avoid all that: cook the beans before you eat them. Cooking beans at high heat (i.e., boiling) denatures most of the anti-nutrients in legumes, rendering them completely or mostly inert. An excess intake of uncooked beans has been shown to stunt growth and damage tissues, but in the modern world, the only ones likely to suffer from this are laboratory rats.

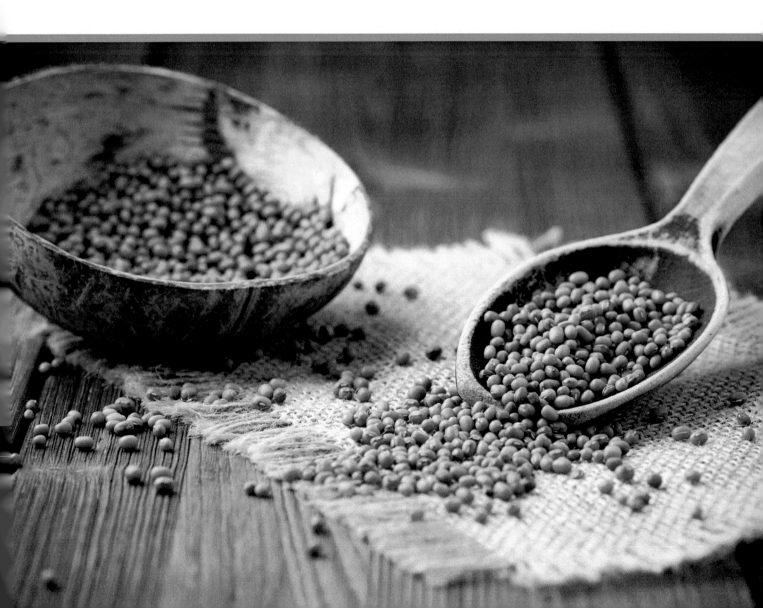

Occasionally concerns are raised about the quality of protein found in legumes. These concerns are generally unfounded unless you plan to devote your diet entirely to beans. Protein quality is a function of how complete the protein is and how readily it is absorbed. A protein molecule is composed of individual amino acids. There are twenty-eight individual amino acids that are assembled in different forms to create all the proteins in our bodies. We can manufacture some of these amino acids internally but require a handful of them in our diet.

Methionine is one such essential amino acid, meaning that humans must get it from their diet and can't make it on their own. Amino acids are the basic building blocks of protein, which make up our muscles, receptors (like the insulin receptor), and enzymes needed for important functions like digestion. A balanced diet including protein from plant and animal sources provides plenty of essential amino acids, but because they lack methionine, beans alone are not able to completely satisfy our nutritional needs. When lab animals are exclusively fed bean diets, they suffer from malnutrition and poor growth as a result. For humans, it is unlikely that this will be relevant unless beans are your only source of protein (which I would not recommend). Once again, it is good not to be a lab rat.

On the bright side, beans also have a number of positive attributes beyond the protein and fiber. Saponins in beans have been postulated to reduce cholesterol and reduce cancer risk, possibly by forming complexes that bind toxins and cholesterol, blocking absorption. Soybeans in particular have even more powerful cholesterol-lowering attributes, discussed in more detail ahead.

Some readers will note that other books referencing the "caveman" diet advise against including legumes in the diet. The argument is that legumes can be harmful to the health if eaten raw, especially if they are a staple of the diet; therefore, it is unlikely that cavemen enjoyed them routinely.

We aren't trying to recreate the caveman diet for posterity's sake but as a template for good health. By returning to our roots we intend to avoid foods that have been introduced to our diet too recently for our bodies to have adapted, especially those that have been associated with poor health.

Legumes have consistently been shown to be an important part of the healthy diet, particularly the well-known, heart-healthy Mediterranean diet. For today's modern cavemen, the benefits of legumes make them an indispensable part of a healthy diet. As we will cover in a later section, legumes such as soy are rich in antioxidants and phytochemicals that lower cholesterol and reduce the risk of cancer and heart disease. In fact, their greater reliance on dietary soy may be one of the reasons that Asian cultures tend to have a lower incidence of heart disease.

But enjoying legumes doesn't mean violating the principles of the ancestral diet; evidence is still ambiguous on whether legumes were part of the caveman diet. Archeological digs in the Middle East have unearthed fossilized legumes right along with pistachios and acorns, suggesting that even before the Agricultural Era legumes had made it onto the ancestral table.

The study of our ancestral diet is one that is clearly still controversial; cavemen unfortunately kept no records, leaving it to researchers to analyze fossilized poop samples and piles of garbage to divine what they ate. Fossilized records leave much to interpretation, and given this uncertainty, it makes sense to give any natural food—especially one with the potential health benefits of legumes—a spot on our dinner tables.

GO NUTS

What would you say if I told you about a snack that is tasty, filling, and could reduce your risk of coronary heart disease by 37% and your risk of sudden cardiac death by almost half? Sounds good, doesn't it?

Yes, nuts really can do all that. The consumption of tree nuts (such as almonds, walnuts, cashews, hazelnuts, and pistachios) and peanuts (technically a legume but with similar health benefits) is associated with significant improvements in cardiovascular health and possibly a reduction in the risk of diabetes. The greatest benefit goes to those who eat 4–5 servings or more per week.

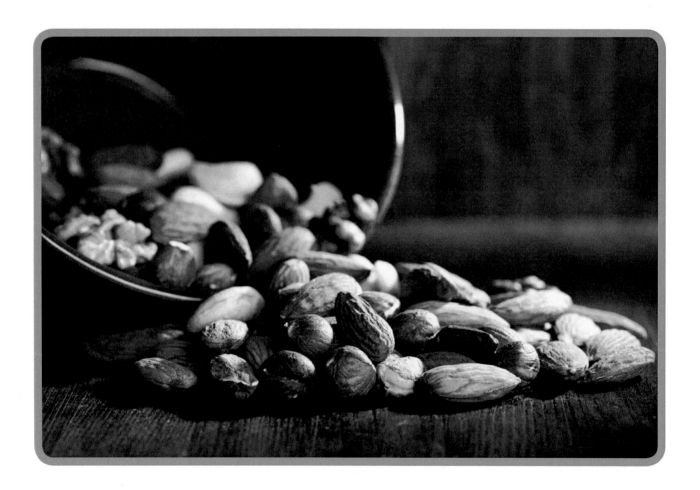

Why are nuts so healthy? It helps to think of nuts and seeds as embryos of the plant world, replete with everything a plant (or you, for that matter) needs to grow up big and strong. They are high in plant sterols, which block absorption of cholesterol in the gut, lowering LDL and total cholesterol. They are high in mono- and poly-unsaturated fats that lower bad cholesterol and raise good cholesterol. And they are packed with protein, fiber, potassium, magnesium, B vitamins, and other micronutrients. Compared to almost every other naturally available food, nuts are about as healthy and complete as you can get.

While all nuts have been shown to improve heart health, there are two that stand out at the head of the class: almonds and walnuts. Walnuts have the highest amount of omega-3 fats among the commonly consumed nuts and almonds have the most fiber. In one clinical trial, walnuts were associated with a 10% reduction in LDL ("bad") cholesterol and almonds with a 13% reduction in LDL cholesterol. In another study, adding almonds to the diet was associated with up to a 9% reduction in LDL. Other nuts, including peanuts, pecans, pistachios, and macadamia nuts, have similar benefits.

How many nuts does it take to lower your cholesterol? Most trials studied anything from 30 to 70 grams of nuts per day, which is equivalent to about 1–2 handfuls. An almond weighs a little over a gram, so you're looking at about 25–60 nuts per day. Thirty almonds provide about 200 calories, which makes for a nice snack between meals. Two snacks a day will get you to the high "dose" studied in trials.

I know what you're thinking: won't eating nuts make me fat? In a word: no.

It is true that nuts have a lot of calories, mostly fat and protein. The good news is that fat and protein are more satiating than carbohydrates; a small handful of nuts fills you up even better than a large muffin. This may be why nuts are generally not associated with weight gain in clinical trials.

Much of the benefit to nuts is in the soft inner shell, so if you are having peanuts or pistachios be sure to eat that part too. Roasted nuts retain their antioxidants and other health benefits. Enjoy them as snack or meal replacements, but avoid salted varieties and try to enjoy them as our ancestors did—raw or roasted; nothing added and nothing taken away.

If roasted almonds aren't your thing, go with walnuts next and other nuts in no particular order after that. Nut flours and butters are okay as long as you watch the amount and make sure that there aren't any ingredients other than nuts. Peanut butter in particular is often packed with emulsifiers, salt, and sugar...no bueno.

All nuts are associated with better cardiovascular health.

---

*Almonds pack the most fiber, while walnuts have
the highest amount of healthy omega-3 fats.*

NATURE'S SWEET TEMPTATIONS

Nature gives us a few delicious sources of pure natural sugars. In the cool Northeastern states, maple trees produce ample quantities of sap that can be distilled into syrup. The spiny agave plant in the arid Southwestern deserts contains a deliciously sweet nectar. And of course the sugarcane, harvested in the tropics, gives us table sugar.

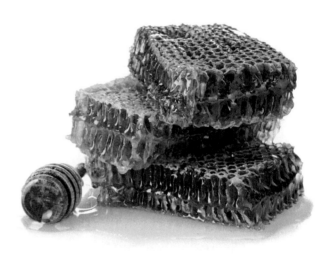

While these sugars are certainly natural, they aren't necessarily healthy. It's tempting to think we could craft an all-natural diet of maple syrup-covered sweet potatoes, but that would just make you the first caveman to develop diabetes and heart disease. Natural sugars still have plenty of sucrose and fructose that play havoc with your metabolism. Dumping loads of sucrose into your system drives up insulin levels, promoting diabetes and weight gain. Excess fructose does not trigger insulin production but instead travels directly to the liver and is either burned as fuel or converted directly into triglycerides for storage in fat cells. When fructose is ingested in large quantities (think about a 40 oz. super-sized Coke with 137 grams of high-fructose corn syrup), the liver cranks up the triglyceride production. These triglycerides end up in your abdominal cavity as fat, lining the organs and giving your belly a nice round look.

Nowhere in nature are you going to find 137 grams of fructose, which is one of the most compelling reasons to stick with our ancestral diet. A tablespoon of honey has just 17 grams of fructose, for example. A tablespoon here or there isn't a problem, but once you start racking up the tablespoons you'd better reach for your elastic pants.

Keep in mind our guiding rule—think like a modern-day caveman or -woman. Honey, agave nectar, sugarcane, and maple syrup were hardly dietary staples prior to agriculture and industry making them readily available. Besides, if you wanted honey back in the prehistoric days, you'd have to grapple an entire colony of bees before you could plunder their honey. In the arid desert you'd have to work your way around the spines of an agave plant before enjoying the sweet nectar inside. Forget trying to get maple syrup—who wants to dig into a maple tree with a rock and a stick just to eat sap? Think like a caveman and you'll manage just fine.

Enjoy natural sugars such as honey,
agave, and maple syrup sparingly, if at all.

EVEN CAVEMEN HAVE TO LIVE A LITTLE

Just to be clear, we aren't attempting to overly glamorize the caveman lifestyle; our ancestral diet is simply a clean slate devoid of the modern foods that make someone else a boatload of money while tempting us into the waiting arms of the pharmaceutical companies. Since we aren't *really* cavemen, we should definitely take into consideration some basics of modern life that are worth including in our diet right from the beginning. The list of "modern" foods to add to our menu is extremely short so we can cover them before we begin our Challenges.

NOW YOU'RE COOKING WITH OIL

Cooking with oil is a relatively recent innovation, dating back to around 3000 BC. Despite the resourcefulness of this invention, it was over four millennia later that someone thought to heat up a batch of oil and drop in a sliced potato. After that milestone it took only another 150 years for French fries to go mainstream.

The first oils were mechanically pressed from olives or other oil-rich plants. Extra virgin labels tell you which oils are still processed this way and retain the most nutrients from the original plant. On the other hand, many oils that do not carry the extra virgin label have been chemically processed and stripped of everything but the fat component. Many of these processed oils are very recent additions to our diet. For example, corn oil was first commercialized in the 1960s, barely half a century ago.

To stay true to our whole food, natural, evolutionary diet we would ideally avoid cooking oils completely. We could enjoy avocados, nuts, and olives whole without squeezing the oil out of them. This would certainly lower your calorie intake and help you stay slim and healthy.

While this is a reasonable and healthy choice, many of us would like to continue to enjoy the variety of cooking options that oils give us. For example, I know that my wife gets pretty tired of my burning chicken on the grill and looks forward to breaking out the fry pans from time to time. While this does add calories, if we choose our cooking oil wisely we can actually improve our health by emphasizing healthy fats in our diet and avoiding the unhealthy ones.

When shopping for oil, the usual choices we'll come across include corn, vegetable, canola, and olive oils. Some grocers will stock specialty oils such as coconut, walnut, or even avocado as well, although these latter oils may be too expensive for regular use.

It should come as no surprise that olive oil is the best choice for cooking. Olive oil has long been associated with good health and is an important part of the heart-healthy Mediterranean diet. Olive oil is rich in monounsaturated fats that raise good cholesterol and reduce bad cholesterol. While we could make a case for using certain other oils, such as coconut or avocado, I will skip to the punch line and tell you that unless you have a compelling reason otherwise, I would stick with olive oil for most cooking applications. Read the second Challenge for more on this topic.

Olive oil is the best choice for cooking.

Anyone who's gone shopping for their own cooking oil can tell you that olive oil isn't the cheapest option out there. Plentiful supply (i.e., government subsidies) makes corn and vegetable oils attractive on a purely financial basis, so these are found in many restaurant or processed foods. Don't succumb to temptation when ordering out—steer clear of anything deep fried.

Is olive oil a bad choice for high-heat cooking?

Aside from flavor, two concerns that often come up when discussing cooking oils are the smoke point and the amount of oxidation that occurs when cooking.

The smoke point is the temperature at which the oil begins to smoke with heating. The smoke itself is a sign that the fatty acids in the oil are breaking down and becoming volatile, hence the acrid smoke that arises. Most oils have similar smoke points around 350–450°F, which is plenty hot enough for cooking. While there is a range of temperatures among oils, the differences are not great enough to warrant making a choice on cooking oil based on smoke points. That being said, extra virgin olive oil may smoke earlier than other oils because it is not chemically processed to remove little fragments of olive that may still be in the solution. These little olive pieces will burn first, causing the oil to smoke before reaching the true smoke point of the oil itself. The bottom line is that olive oil can hold roughly the same temperatures as most other oils for domestic cooking.

This brings us to the topic of oxidation. All oils will interact with oxygen in the air when heated, and that interaction generates free radicals that are harmful to our health. This topic will come up again and again throughout this book. The amount of oxidation is a function of two things: the type of oil and the amount of antioxidants in the oil. The saturated fats in coconut oil and the monounsaturated fats in olive and avocado oils are most resistant to oxidative damage. Extra virgin olive oil has the added benefit of antioxidants in the oil that protect both the oil and us from any free radicals that might be created in the cooking process.

You can safely cook with olive oil at home but don't leave it on heat too long. One study showed that after frying one batch of potatoes in olive oil fully 80% of the antioxidants were retained in the food and oil, while only 20% remained after three to four batches. Cooking each batch of food in a fresh pan of oil is the best way to limit the amount of oxidation that occurs. Also, since only oil that is in contact with air will oxidize, deep-frying actually involves less oxidation than pan-frying. The same study mentioned above also showed that foods that were deep fried retained significantly more antioxidants than those that were pan-fried. It might not help you trim your waistline but at least it will save you from a bit of free radicals.

If you tire of olive oil, avocado or coconut oils are reasonable alternatives. The saturated fats in coconut oil are even more resistant to oxidation than the monounsaturated fats in olive and avocado oils. Also, since coconut oil is a solid at room temperature it has a texture suitable for baked goods, such as almond-flour muffins. Avocado has a similar fatty acid profile to olive oil but may not have the same antioxidants and has not been studied as extensively as olive oil for its potential health benefits. We'll cover these topics again in Challenges #2 and #5.

STAYING AWAKE AND STAYING HEALTHY

Caffeine is a naturally-occurring stimulant found in plants such as tea, coffee, cocoa, guarana, and yerba mate, among others. Caffeine is a benign indulgence–it has not been associated with any long-term adverse health consequences when consumed in moderation. Studies have shown that caffeine enhances attention, reaction time, and thought processing, none of which should shock anyone who has pulled an all-nighter or two in college. While a cup of coffee may transiently increase your blood pressure, chronic caffeine intake (the same amount every day) has not been shown to have a lasting effect on blood pressures. Furthermore, daily caffeine intake is not associated with any increase in cardiovascular risk and may even reduce your risk of diabetes. Caffeine ingestion is also associated with a lower risk of dementia with aging. If you are already enjoying caffeinated beverages there is no reason to change but keep your consumption to a moderate amount.

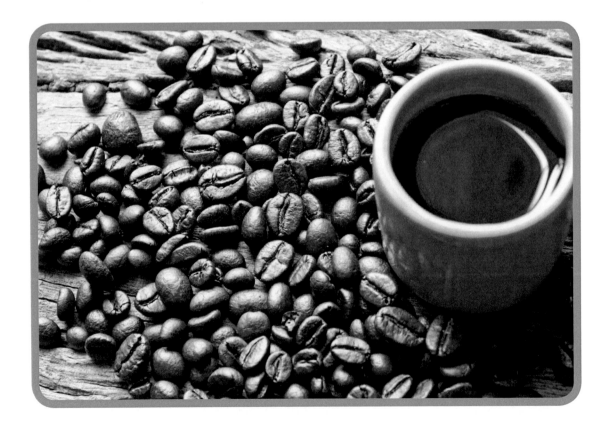

Where you get your caffeine definitely matters. Green tea, black tea, and coffee have antioxidant benefits and have been shown to reduce the risk of diabetes and heart disease. We all know that sugary beverages and sodas are no good for us, so it should be obvious that we would want to avoid these when looking for a buzz. Diet sodas as well should be approached with caution, as consumption of diet sodas tends to promote weight gain. Moreover, the acid and sodium in sodas promote osteoporosis and high blood pressure, as we will see in later chapters. So stick to tea and coffee, black or unsweetened if you can tolerate it.

TAKE TWO DRINKS AND CALL ME IN THE MORNING

While alcohol is a relatively new addition to the human diet, it does have measurable benefits when enjoyed in moderation. Moderate alcohol intake (1 drink per day for women, 1–2 for men) is associated with increased HDL (good) cholesterol and better overall cardiovascular health. Any alcohol will give you this effect, regardless of the source; however, giving some thought to your choice of libation is worthwhile. Red wine, covered in detail in Challenge #5, is rich in antioxidants not found in any other alcoholic beverage, including white wine. Sugary cocktails and beers are high in calories and sugars and should be avoided. Spirits are low in calories; a vodka and soda has only about 40–60 calories per serving. If you choose not to enjoy red wine, stick to low-calorie spirits and avoid the sugary drinks and beer. It's tough to get healthy if these comprise any part of your diet.

If you are a teetotaler today you need not start imbibing just for your health. If you are already drinking, just limit yourself to 1–2 drinks per day. If you find this hard, talk to your doctor.

Caffeine and alcohol in moderation are beneficial to your health.

That's it for the cheats. I know what you're thinking—you expected a few more, didn't you? The answer to this one is no, at least not now. The beauty of the ancestral diet is its simplicity. Remember our guiding principle: if it wasn't around a million years ago, don't eat it. Don't make life complicated by asking a lot of "but what about X?" questions. Do that often enough and you'll be back where you started. Limit starchy vegetables; enjoy some olive oil, caffeine, and alcohol in moderation. That's it. Keeping it simple allows you to stay focused and get the results that you came here for: better health and fewer medications.

Now it's time to head to the kitchen and start putting all this good knowledge into practice eating like a modern day hunter-gatherer.

Don't just eat like a caveman, eat like a Mediterranean caveman.

The countries circling the Mediterranean have traditionally had a lower risk of heart disease than the rest of the developed world. This has long been attributed to the diet of Mediterranean cultures, which is rich in many of the all-natural foods we have just learned about. For example, the Mediterranean diet includes an emphasis on olive oil, nuts, fruits, vegetables, legumes, fish, and white meat.

As we discussed earlier in the section on meat, the Mediterranean diet was studied in a large trial of over 7,000 people to see if it truly did lead to a reduction in heart attacks. This trial, published in THE NEW ENGLAND JOURNAL OF MEDICINE, showed that among people at high risk of heart disease (including people who are overweight and have high cholesterol, blood sugars, and blood pressures), eating a Mediterranean diet was associated with a 30% reduction in heart attack and other cardiovascular events (such as stroke or death) when compared to those eating a more typical Western diet.

The table below illustrates the basic elements of the Mediterranean diet studied in this trial. We will learn more about these specific foods as we go through the Challenges, but even now it is worth trying to incorporate them into your caveman diet. Enjoy these "power foods" as often as you can, but keep the wine in moderation.

The Mediterranean Caveman Diet

Encouraged	Anount Recommended	Discouraged	Amount Recommended
Olive Oil	4 tbls/day	Red meat	< 1 serving per day
Nuts	3 servings per week	Soda	< 1 drink per day
Fruits	3 servings per day	Baked goods	< 3 servings per week
Vegetables	2 servings per day	Spread fats	< 1 serving per day
Fish	3 servings per week		
Lecumes	3 servings per week		
Sofrito	2 servings per week		
White Meat	Substitute for red meat		
Wine	1 drink per day		

Source: Estruch, et al. NEJM. 2013.

Paul F., age 68

Dr. Dave's program saved my life, literally. I'd climbed the career ladder for forty years; in my mid-sixties I looked as if I were nine months pregnant, had no muscle tone, and was taking way too many medications. Twenty-five years of smoking had left me wheezing and coughing after even minimal exertion, so I rarely attempted even that. When we met, he took one look at my chart and proceeded to convince me that I was on a path that led to disaster, no matter how much I tried to kid myself otherwise. It wasn't long before I was talked out of my inertia and agreed to give his group a try.

I hadn't dieted or exercised in years, but Dr. Dave pushed me to work hard at getting results. Not long after starting to work out I got lightheaded and almost passed out during my workout. Dr. Dave ordered a stress test, which I passed. He didn't believe it and ordered another one. This time the results showed that I had a serious blockage in the arteries leading to the heart. My heart wasn't squeezing hard enough during exercise to push blood to my brain; that's why I was getting lightheaded in the gym. One minute I was totally fine (or so I thought) and the next minute they were telling me that I needed to have heart surgery. I eventually got eleven stents placed in my coronary arteries, and thankfully I was in and out of the hospital in only a few days. Eight weeks later I was back in the workouts alongside the rest of the guys.

I now have a renewed zest for life that I never thought possible at this age. I feel as if I've evolved from sixty-eight to fifty years old. With Dr. Dave's program I have transformed from "old fat guy" to "old fit guy" in eleven months. I'm forty-five pounds lighter and have reduced my waist size from 40 to 34, with eating habits that are satisfying and an exercise regimen that is demanding but fun. I've met some great guys and I look forward to every workout. The opportunity to work out with people in your own age group is unique and inclusive.

The physical changes are dramatic and people who haven't seen me in a few months are constantly taken aback by how I look. I've just gotten a bunch of new suits tailored to my trimmer physique: from borderline portly to trim fit! Most importantly, I no longer worry about my health or my ability to take care of my wife and family. One year after my heart scare I passed my stress test with flying colors. I'm back!

I encourage you to join us—regardless of your age, gender, or fitness. There's a place for you here.

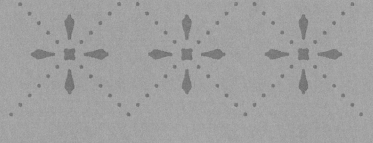

PART III

THE CHALLENGES

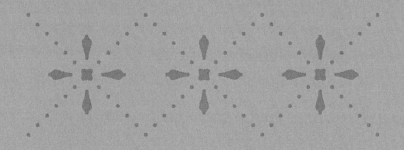

CHALLENGE #1: EAT LIKE A CAVEMAN

Start your diet with a clean slate

SO NOW THAT WE'VE LEARNED THE BASICS OF THE ANCESTRAL-BASED DIET, IT'S TIME TO GIVE IT A TRY. Our first Challenge is to clear our plates of the trappings of Western culture and go back, way back, to our dietary roots. Forget about bread (10–30,000 years ago), ice cream (2,000 years ago), and pasta (less than 1,000 years ago). We are going to follow one simple rule from this point forward: if it wasn't around one million years ago, don't eat it. That one simple rule will carry you through every restaurant, shopping trip, and lunch meeting. It makes every diet decision so easy, even a caveman could do it.

This simplicity is one of the most compelling aspects of our ancestral-based diet. Think of other diets you may have tried: South Beach, Atkins, Zone, or even just low-carb or low-fat diets. All have relatively complex rules to follow—what is good and what is bad? Here we are going to stick with one easy and common sense rule that will serve as the foundation for everything that is to come.

It is important to get this one right. Take your time, learn some recipes, and have some fun filling your plate with new foods. Items that were once a garnish or side may become the main dish. You may find that you are trying new foods that you haven't really given much thought in the past. Go back to my words of advice and hunker down for a month or two of really getting this under your belt.

By now you should have a grasp for what foods to be thinking about as you embark on your first days as a hunter-gatherer. If there's any doubt, refer to the table below for a quick look at what to enjoy and what to avoid.

AS MUCH AS YOU WANT	MODERATION	AVOID ALTOGETHER
Low GI foods Green veggies Legumes Lean meats Fish and seafood Nuts Fruits	Moderate GI foods Sweet potatoes Seeds Healthy oils	High GI foods White potatoes Wheat and grains Rice Natural sugars Processed foods Corn and soy oils

Next we'll learn some new staple foods for breakfast, lunch, and dinner. Most Next we'll learn some new staple foods for breakfast, lunch, and dinner. Most of us are used to cereal, oatmeal, or yogurt for breakfast, sandwiches and chips for lunch, and some rice, pasta, or bread with dinner. As we get rid of these we are going to need to fill our pantries and our stomachs with some new foods in order to make this work. In this first Challenge, feel free to really enjoy the variety of foods that are found in nature. Don't worry about quantity—pile your plate high. Remember my advice from the beginning and reread it before you begin. If you are surprised to see that steaks are back on the list, go out and get some. You will be giving up some old treats so be sure to enjoy some new ones.

You may find that some additional reading helps you understand the nuances of the diet and get some recipe ideas. The hunter-gatherer diet we've discussed is often called the Paleolithic Diet (or Paleo for short), in reference to the Paleolithic Era, which preceded the Agricultural Era and spans the most recent chapter of our evolution to modern man. I've given you the basics of this diet, but I'd encourage you to explore the works of others to gain more understanding as well as more recipe ideas. When you look for recipes, be sure that they are consistent with the guidelines that I am giving you.

Challenge #1: Your first Challenge is to adhere to a hunter-gatherer diet until you are able to maintain it strictly for at least two weeks. Begin a food log, writing down everything you eat with the exception of calorie-free beverages.

A note on the recipes in this book:

I enjoy learning new recipes and am always looking for vegetarian or Paleo recipes that can help get us off medications and on the road to health and longevity. Each of the Challenges is followed by a handful of my favorite recipes and suggestions from current members to help you get started.

The recipes in this book are ones that I have come across in my own research and have been tweaked to remove any elements that lead to poor health (e.g., excess salt and carbohydrates). Many were contributed by my friends and patients. Where possible I have given specific credit to the original authors of the recipes from which these are derived. In other cases, the original provenance is unknown or long forgotten; however, I humbly give credit to all of the chefs whose work makes this collection possible.

In addition to this book, these online resources are also a rich trove of recipes that are often consistent with our guidelines. Explore these and others as you embark on your culinary adventures:

- www.paleomg.com
- www. simply-vegetarian.com
- www. againstallgrain.com
- www. whole9life.com
- www. theclothesmakethegirl.com/wellfed

"EAT LIKE A CAVEMAN" RECIPES

BREAKFAST

WITH A DAY JOB AND A FAMILY TO CARE FOR, THE ONLY "BREAK" IN MY BREAKFAST IS A CHAOTIC BREAK FOR THE DOOR. Unfortunately, this means that if my breakfast isn't ready to go, I'm likely to go hungry and that's definitely no fun. Furthermore, my wife has no intention of getting up at 4:30 am to make a nice breakfast, and who could blame her? Rather than risk being hungry and cranky all day, I usually make breakfast ahead of time either at night or on weekends then stick it in the fridge for a quick grab out the door. Frittatas, egg scrambles, or pancakes are all great reheated on the go.

EGG SCRAMBLES AND FRITTATAS

One of my favorite breakfast staples is too simple to warrant a recipe: eggs scrambled with vegetables. Just sauté some chopped veggies in olive oil for a few minutes then drop in the eggs. Divide into containers and keep in the fridge for a couple of days' worth of breakfasts. Leftovers from the night before make for great breakfasts, either mixed with eggs or by themselves.

Remember to keep to only about one egg yolk per day and make up the remainder with egg whites. Keep the below ingredients on hand and pull from each column to make an endless variety of scrambles, omelets, or frittatas for serving and storing.

EGGS	VEGETABLES	MEATS	SPICES
Omega-3 eggs Egg whites	Broccoli Cauliflower Peppers Onions Zucchini Spinach	Chicken Pork Beef Salmon Shrimp Scallops	White pepper Black pepper Salt-free seasoning blend Garlic Oregano Basil

SCRAMBLE

1) Heat olive oil on medium heat.
2) Sauté vegetables and spices for a few minutes until tender.
3) Add eggs and precooked meat, scramble, and serve.

FRITTATA

1) Preheat oven to 350°F.
2) Sauté vegetables and spices in olive oil.
3) Whisk eggs in bowl.
4) Wait until vegetables are tender then add the spinach, meat, and eggs.
5) When eggs start to firm up around the edges, place in oven until center is firm, about 20 min.
6) Cut into 4 servings and place in containers for easy breakfast during the week.

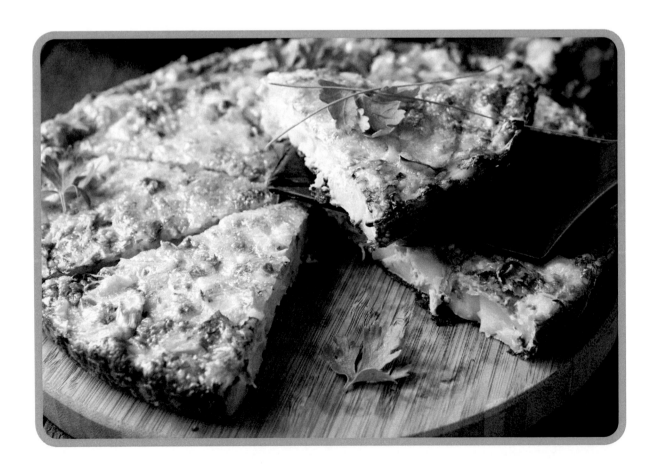

The most important meal of the day

Isn't that what your mother told you about breakfast? Clearly, she didn't realize how busy you are…rushing out of the house with just a bite of toast and a cup of coffee. You grab a muffin around midmorning, and then finally eat something around lunch if you can. The good news is that you must be losing weight by saving a meal at breakfast, right?

Unfortunately, the answer is no. While skipping breakfast is not exactly a hot topic at the World Health Organization or the National Institutes of Health, it has been studied enough to confirm what your stomach is probably already telling you…skipping breakfast is not good for you. Check out these findings from breakfast studies around the world:

- Women who skipped breakfast were shown to have increased total calories for theday, increased insulin resistance (the first sign of diabetes), and higher total and LDLcholesterol.

- Adolescents who skip breakfast may be less likely to eat fruits and vegetables later in the day (go figure).

- In Philadelphia, aptitude tests showed that children who skipped breakfast were just as smart but not as happy as kids who do eat breakfast.

- In Poland, research suggested that skipping breakfast was even more closely as-sociated with weight gain than was the choice of foods during the rest of the day.

- An American study showed that skipping breakfast worsened problem-solving skills.

- To top it all off, a worldwide meta-analysis of over 93,000 study subjects showed a 75% higher chance of obesity in those who skipped breakfast.

So don't skimp on breakfast. Instead, treat it like what it is: the most important meal of the day. Take the time at night or in the morning to prepare a healthy breakfast and have it on the go if need be. You'll probably find that you have more energy and sharper faculties, make better food choices, lose more weight, and feel better as a result.

SMOOTHIE RECIPES

In a pinch nothing beats a smoothie in the morning. Some people like to juice their veggies, but then you lose a lot of the fiber and have more mess to clean up. Invest in a decent blender capable of pureeing veggies until smooth, and then go have some fun. There's no wrong way to make a smoothie so play around with some recipes and enjoy!

VEGGIE-BERRY PROTEIN SMOOTHIE

2 cups of soy milk
One cup of spinach or kale leaves (any green vegetable)

½ cup berries
½ banana
1 scoop protein powder

- Blend, add water to desired consistency.

5AM PROTEIN SMOOTHIE

1 scoop protein powder
2 cups of soy milk
2–3 tsp. instant coffee

2 tbsp. cocoa
½ banana

- Blend, add water to desired consistency.

SPINACH LIME SMOOTHIE

2 tbsp. lime juice
2 cups of spinach leaves, chopped
1 cup of frozen mango or berries

1 cup of green grapes
½ cup water

- Add water to blender, followed by other ingredients. Blend until smooth.

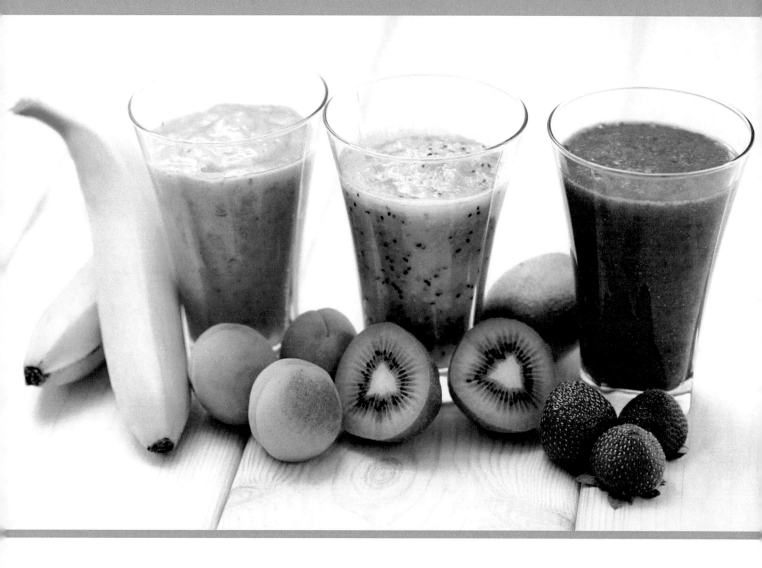

Who says cavemen can't have pancakes? These recipes satisfy your craving for pancakes, waffles, or muffins in the morning and offer a healthy alternative to a carbohydrate-laden, flour-based American-style breakfast. The best part is that these treats keep well and can be enjoyed for days after making. Make a stack of pancakes on Sunday and put them in the fridge for a quick snack or breakfast on the go.

PUMPKIN PANCAKES

¼ cup pumpkin puree
2 tbsp. almond or soy milk
2 eggs
1 tsp. agave nectar
1 tbsp. vanilla extract
2 tbsp. coconut flour

½ cup almond flour
1 tsp. cinnamon
¼ tsp. ground ginger
⅛ tsp. ground cloves
2 tsp. olive oil

- Mix wet ingredients thoroughly.
- Whisk all of the dry ingredients separately.
- Mix wet and dry together.
- Spoon or pour onto a skillet at low-medium heat (smaller pancakes will flip more easily).
- Cook about 5 minutes on each side.

EASY PEASY PANCAKES (ADAPTED FROM PALEOPARENTS.COM)

2 cups almond flour

1 banana, chunked into small pieces

4 omega-3 enriched eggs

⅔ cup light soy milk or almond milk

1 tsp. vanilla extract

1 tbsp. olive oil

- Blend banana, eggs, and milk until smooth.
- Mix in the dry ingredients.
- Bring a pan to medium heat, coat with olive oil.
- Form small, easy-to-flip pancakes with batter. Smaller is easier.
- Cook until bottom is golden brown and edges are starting to firm. The pancake should be forming small bubbles in the center.
- Flip and brown the other side. Remove when evenly browned.

PERFECT PANCAKES

1½ cups of almond flour

½ cup coconut milk

4 eggs

1 tsp. sodium-free baking powder

1 tsp. cinnamon

1 tsp. vanilla extract

- Combine dry ingredients and mix thoroughly.
- Beat eggs and mix with wet ingredients.
- Blend wet and dry ingredients.
- Heat skillet to medium-low, form small pancakes with batter.
- Flip when brown, about 2–3 minutes for each side.

APPLE EGG MUFFINS

3 large green apples, chopped
3 tbsp. warm water
2 tsp. cinnamon

9 egg whites, plus 2 yolks
1 tsp. vanilla extract
1–2 tbsp. coconut flour

- Preheat oven to 350°F.
- Sauté apples, water, and cinnamon until the apples are soft.
- Whisk eggs and coconut flour.
- Add apples to egg mixture.
- Pour into lined muffin tins.
- Bake for 30 min. or until a toothpick inserted in the center comes out clean.

"OATMEAL"

2 eggs
½ cup unsweetened shredded coconut

2 dates, finely chopped
½ tsp. cinnamon

- Place all ingredients in saucepan.
- Whisk while on low.
- Keep whisking until mixture starts to thicken.
- Serve when at desired consistency.

ALMOND FLOUR MUFFINS

2½ cups almond flour
¾ tsp. sodium-free baking powder
3 large eggs
⅓ cup mashed, ripe banana
2 tbsp. honey
2 tbsp. coconut oil, melted

1 tsp. white vinegar
1 tsp. vanilla extract
1 tsp. cinnamon
Blueberries (alternatives include cacao nibs or chopped walnuts)

- Preheat oven to 350°F.
- Line 10 cups in a standard 12-cup muffin tin with paper or foil liners.
- Whisk dry ingredients in mixing bowl.

- Combine wet ingredients separately and mix thoroughly.
- Add the wet ingredients to the dry ingredients, stirring until blended.
- Fold in berries.
- Divide batter evenly among muffin tins.
- Bake for 14 to 18 minutes until set at the centers and golden brown at the edges.
- Remove and allow to cool before removing from tins.
- Remove muffins from tin.

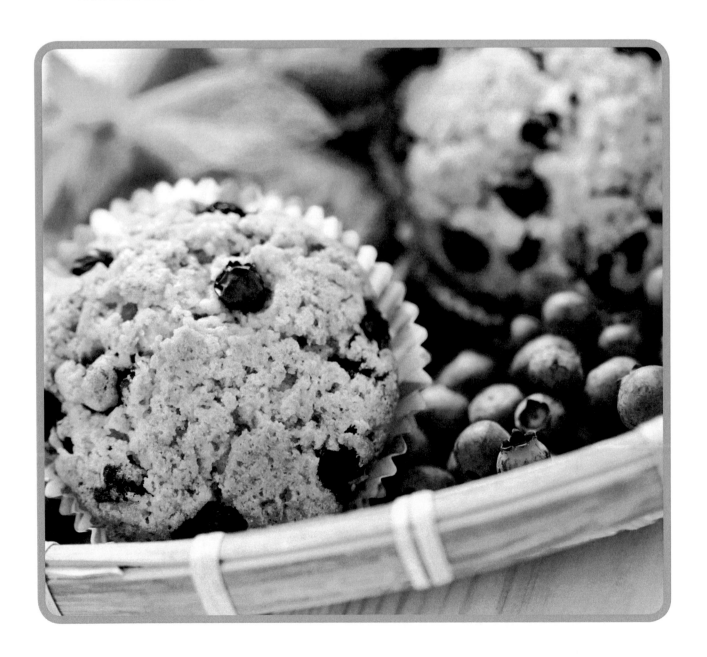

BANANA BREAD MUFFINS (ADAPTED FROM LACY YOUNG & ROB WOLF)

1½ cup almond flour

2 tbsp. ground flaxseed

1 tsp. cinnamon

¼ tsp. sodium-free baking powder

Pinch of nutmeg

2 very ripe bananas, mashed

2 omega-3 eggs

1 tbsp. honey

1 tbsp. olive oil or coconut oil

½ tsp. vanilla extract

⅓ cup chopped walnuts or chopped fruit

- Preheat oven to 375°F.
- Sift together dry ingredients and mix well.
- Put wet ingredients (eggs, honey, bananas, oil, vanilla extract, honey) in blender or food processor and blend thoroughly until smooth.
- Mix wet and dry ingredients. Add nuts and/or chopped fruit.
- Spoon into greased muffin tin.
- Baking time is approximately 20 minutes. They are done when a toothpick comes out clean.

For more baked-good recipes including nut flours check out againstallgrain.com

---

Note on baking like a hunter-gatherer

Many recipes you find will call for baking soda, baking powder, or a pinch of salt. Keep in mind that although it doesn't sound like much, one teaspoon of baking soda has 1,200 milligrams (mg) of sodium—enough for your entire day without eating one more bite of anything. Baking powder has a little less than 500 mg per teaspoon, while a teaspoon of table salt has a whopping 2,300 mg of sodium. So remember that a little baking soda or salt goes a long way in your baking.

My recommendation is to try each recipe without the added sodium. Baked goods may come out a little more dense than otherwise, but you may find it tolerable and certainly tasty enough. Another trick is to use club soda in place of water or quick-rise baker's yeast in place of the baking powder or sodium.

LUNCHES, DINNERS, SNACKS & SIDES

PASTA WITHOUT PASTA

Pasta is one of those foods with which many of us have a long-standing love affair. As with any serious relationship, breaking up is hard to do. Instead of getting depressed about our loss, let's find some adventure in new experiences. You may not believe it, but squash and zucchini make an excellent substitute for noodles and pair well with many sauces commonly served with pasta.

Spaghetti squash or zucchini can be prepared as substitutes for spaghetti or fettuccini, depending on how you slice or shred them. Buy whatever looks freshest and is in season. The trick is to cook them long enough to be tender but not too tender to hold a sauce. As with pasta, you will develop a knack for it with practice.

To get your slices just right with ease, consider buying a mandolin or julienne slicer. You can find these online or at any kitchen store (e.g., Bed Bath & Beyond).

....

GRILLED CHICKEN AND PEPPERS OVER SPAGHETTI SQUASH

1 spaghetti squash
1 sliced red onion
1–2 bell peppers

1–2 chicken breasts
Olive oil

- To prepare spaghetti squash, pierce a few times with a knife, place on a microwave-safe dish, and heat for 5 min. Turn squash on other side, heat for additional 5 min. Once done, use oven mitt to hold squash while cutting it lengthwise.
- Separately, sauté onions and peppers in olive oil over medium heat until soft. Set aside.
- Slice chicken breasts thinly and add to pan. Cook thoroughly, turning strips when no longer pink.
- Remove from pan when done; toss all cooked ingredients together with spaghetti squash. Add olive oil to taste if tempted.

PESTO SPAGHETTI SQUASH AND SHRIMP

1 large package fresh basil

2–3 cloves garlic

¼ cup walnuts

About ¼ cup extra virgin olive oil, plus 1 tbsp. separated

1 spaghetti squash

12–16 shrimp

1 pint cherry tomatoes, halved

¼ cup pine nuts

- Prepare spaghetti squash as above.
- Place the basil leaves, garlic, and walnuts in food processor and pulse a few times. Leave running while slowly adding olive oil.
- Heat olive oil in pan, add shrimp and cook until almost pink. Add spaghetti squash, pesto, and cherry tomatoes. Garnish with pine nuts.
- You will find that pesto prepared this way will have a richer basil taste without all the parmesan cheese and added salt. After a few bites you'll never go back.

CHICKEN WITH ASPARAGUS PESTO (ADAPTED FROM SLIMSANITY.COM)

1 spaghetti squash

2 chicken breasts

1 pound asparagus, trimmed

2 cups spinach leaves

1 cup basil leaves

4 cloves garlic (less to taste)

4 tbsp. pine nuts or ¼ cup chopped walnuts

1 cup low- or no-sodium chicken broth

Freshly ground pepper

- Prepare spaghetti squash as above.
- Grill chicken according to taste, set aside.
- Chop asparagus into small pieces and sauté in chicken broth over medium heat until soft.
- Remove from heat but do not discard broth.
- Toast pine nuts if desired over low heat in skillet, being careful not to burn them. Remove from heat.
- Transfer about one-third of the chicken broth from skillet along with all other ingredients to food processor.
- Pulse until smoothly blended. Add remaining chicken broth to bring to desired consistency.
- Layer spaghetti squash on plate, followed by chicken, and top with pesto.
- Serve immediately.

. . . .

SPAGHETTI SQUASH WITH VEGETABLES

1 large spaghetti squash
1 bag frozen mixed vegetables
1 bag frozen okra
2–3 cloves garlic, minced

1 cup chopped chicken breast (rotisserie chicken is easiest)
2 tbsp. olive oil

- Prepare spaghetti squash as above.
- Stir-fry garlic and vegetables over medium heat until tender.
- Add spaghetti squash and chicken breast, cook for another 2–3 minutes, tossing frequently.
- Serve immediately.

CROCKPOT RECIPES

A crockpot or slow cooker is a must-have item in your kitchen, especially if you don't have the luxury of spending hours each week on food prep. Furthermore, since you will be cutting way back on your eating out and processed foods, you will want to have plenty of leftovers from every meal you make at home to maximize the return on your time in the kitchen. With a slow cooker your prep time is minimal, and you simply "set it and forget it."

. . . .

CROCKPOT LEMON HERB CHICKEN

2 pounds of boneless chicken breasts
1 lemon, sliced
1 sprig of fresh rosemary
2–3 sprigs of fresh thyme

Handful of Italian flat leaf parsley
3–4 cloves garlic, chopped
¼ cup water

- Place chicken in crockpot and cover with lemon, herbs, and garlic; pour water over the top.
- Cover and cook on low for 8–10 hours.

20-CLOVE GARLIC CHICKEN

3-4 pounds chicken pieces, skin and excess fat removed
1 large onion, sliced
1 tbsp. olive oil
2 tsp. paprika
1 tsp. pepper
20-40 cloves garlic, peeled, but intact

- Place onion slices on the bottom of the crockpot.
- In a large mixing bowl, toss chicken parts with olive oil, paprika, pepper, and all of the garlic cloves. It helps to boil the cloves for 1-2 minutes to soften them before peeling; it's a lot of garlic to peel otherwise. Alternatively, use them unpeeled and simply apply a little pressure to extract the garlic after serving.
- Pour ingredients into slow cooker, on top of the onion (do not add water).
- Cover and cook on low for 6-8 hours or on high for 4-6 hours.
- Serve with vegetables of your choosing.

BALSAMIC CROCKPOT SHORT RIBS

2-3 pounds bone-in, grass-fed short ribs
1 tbsp. coconut oil
1 15 oz. can plain tomato sauce (no salt)
½ cup balsamic vinegar
4 dates (whole)
6 cloves garlic, smashed

- Brown ribs in coconut oil.
- Place the rest of the ingredients in crock pot; place ribs in sauce.
- Cover and cook for 4-6 hours on high, or until meat is tender.

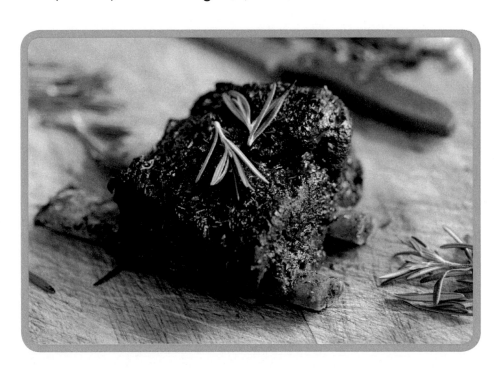

. . . .

CROCKPOT BEEF BRISKET

2–3 pounds grass-fed beef brisket
Mrs. Dash seasoning blend
6 cloves garlic, smashed and peeled

1 large yellow onion
2 cups water

- Slice onion thinly and layer on bottom of crockpot.
- Add garlic cloves, whole.
- Season beef liberally with Mrs. Dash seasoning and place on top of onions, fat side up.
- Pour water over the beef. It will not cover the meat.
- Cook on low for 8–10 hours. Serve *au jus* accompanied by onions and garlic.

OVEN AND STOVETOP RECIPES

Break out your baking trays and frying pans for some meals that will get dinner on the table in a jiffy.

. . . .

STEAMED CLAMS IN WHITE WINE SAUCE

6 dozen fresh clams
3 tbsp. olive oil
4 cloves garlic, chopped
1 large onion, chopped

1 cup white wine
2 cups clam juice or water
Chopped parsley leaves
Salt-free seasoning blend

- Wash the clams thoroughly and remove any blemishes.
- Heat oil in a large saucepan (with a cover) over medium heat.
- Add garlic and onion and cook until translucent.
- Add the wine and simmer for 1–2 minutes.
- Add the clams and clam juice (or water) and cover the pan for about 10 minutes until the clams open.
- Discard any clams that do not open. Distribute clams among serving bowls.
- Season the juices in the pan to make a sauce. Pour the sauce over the clams, garnish with parsley.

STEAMED CLAMS IN SPICY BROTH (ADAPTED FROM MARIO BATALI)

3 tbsp. extra virgin olive oil
1 red onion, thinly sliced
4 cloves garlic, thinly sliced
4 scallions, thinly sliced
4 pounds clams
1 cup tomato puree

1 cup dry white wine
2 tsp. red pepper flakes
1 cup chopped fresh basil
½ cup chopped fresh chives
½ cup fresh oregano leaves

- Wash the clams thoroughly and remove any blemishes.
- Heat oil in large skillet over medium-high heat. Add onions, scallions, and garlic.
- Cook about 5 minutes, stirring occasionally.
- Add clams, tomato puree, wine, and red pepper.
- Bring to boil, reduce heat to medium, cover, and cook until clams open.
- Discard any clams that do not open.
- Uncover pan and add herbs; toss to combine.
- Divide clams among bowls and pour remaining broth over top.

SEAFOOD IN SPICY BROTH (ADAPTED FROM GIADA DE LAURENTIIS)

¼ cup olive oil
5 cloves garlic, minced
1 bay leaf
1 tsp. dried crushed red pepper
1 cup dry white wine
1 28 oz. can diced tomatoes

24 littleneck clams, scrubbed (about 2½ pounds)
24 mussels, debearded (1½ pounds)
20 large shrimp, peeled, deveined, and butterflied (1 pound)
½ cup torn fresh basil leaves

- Heat oil in heavy large pot over medium heat.
- Add garlic, bay leaf, and crushed red pepper.
- Sauté until garlic is tender, about 1 minute.
- Add wine and bring to boil.
- Add tomatoes.
- Simmer until the tomatoes begin to break down, about 5-8 minutes.
- Stir in clams, cook covered for 5 minutes.
- Stir in mussels, cook until clams and mussels open, about 5 more minutes.
- Using tongs, transfer open shellfish to 4-5 serving bowls and discard any unopened shellfish.

- Add shrimp and basil to remaining broth.
- Simmer until shrimp are cooked through, about 1–2 minutes.
- Divide the shrimp and broth among the bowls.
- Serve and enjoy!

CHICKEN PICCATA (ADAPTED FROM PALEO CLIPBOARD)

1½ pounds boneless, skinless chicken breasts, butterflied
Ground black pepper to taste
¼ cup almond flour
¼ cup arrowroot powder
1 small white onion, chopped
2 cloves garlic, chopped

¼ cup olive oil or coconut oil
½ cup fresh squeezed lemon juice
¾ cup low- or no-sodium chicken broth
¼ cup capers, drained and rinsed
⅓ cup fresh parsley, chopped (plus more for garnish, optional)

- Mix the almond flour and arrowroot powder together in medium-sized bowl. Dredge the chicken breasts in the mixture and set aside.
- Sauté garlic and onion in half the olive oil over medium heat.
- Add chicken breasts and cook for about 3 minutes on each side.
- Add the lemon juice, chicken broth, capers, black pepper, and fresh parsley to the pan and allow to reduce for about 3 minutes.
- Return the chicken to the pan and reduce heat to low.
- Cover and simmer for about 5 minutes.
- Transfer to serving dish, garnish with parsley, and serve.

MUSHROOM MEATBALLS AND TOMATO SAUCE (ADAPTED FROM SARAH FRAGOSO)

1 pound diced mushrooms, any variety
1 pound ground beef
2 cloves garlic, minced
½ cup Italian parsley, minced
2 egg yolks
1 tsp. black pepper
1–2 tbsp. coconut oil

1 28 oz. can Marzano tomatoes
3 tbsp. extra virgin olive oil
1 cup fresh basil, chopped
Black pepper to taste

- Combine the mushrooms, beef, garlic, Italian parsley, egg yolks, and pepper in a large mixing bowl.
- Shape mixture into meatballs about 1–2 inches thick.
- In a large sauté pan, heat the coconut oil over medium-high heat.
- Add the meatballs to the hot pan and brown them on all sides.
- Remove the browned meatballs from the pan and set them aside.
- Add tomatoes, olive oil, basil, and pepper to pan.
- Bring to a boil, then reduce to simmer, stirring occasionally.
- Add the meatballs to the simmering sauce, cover, and simmer over low heat for 15–20 minutes or until the meatballs are cooked all the way through.

SEARED SCALLOPS

1–2 pounds scallops
2 tbsp. coconut oil

Pepper or other seasonings
Add oil to pan over high heat

- Add scallops, sear until cooked through about ⅛ inch then flip and cook other side evenly.
- The center of the scallop should be translucent when done.
- Remove from pan, season to taste, and serve.

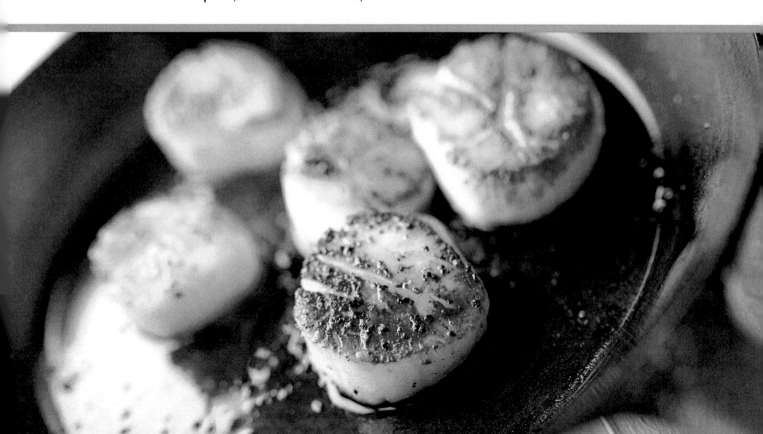

. . . .

NO-SALT BRINED CHICKEN

2 chicken breasts

2 bay leaves

1 tbsp. whole pepper corns

1 tbsp. whole cumin seeds

1 tbsp. whole coriander seeds

2–3 cloves garlic, crushed

- Combine in a gallon-sized zip bag, add water to cover chicken.
- Let sit for 3–24 hours.
- Grill, pan-fry, or bake at 350°F until cooked thoroughly.

. . . .

SECO DE POLLO

2–3 pounds skinless chicken breasts, thighs, or legs, bone in or bone out

2 tbsp. olive oil

1 large onion

1–2 bell peppers

1 large tomato

3 cloves garlic

12 oz. water

Cumin and white pepper to taste

Fresh cilantro leaves for garnish

- Pulse vegetables in food processor until pureed.
- Heat oil in a large pot.
- Season chicken and add to pot, brown on all sides.
- Remove chicken to a plate and set aside.
- Add more oil if needed, turn heat to medium. Transfer vegetables to pan and sauté until soft and onions are translucent.
- Return the chicken to the saucepan, along with the water.
- Simmer on medium-low for around 25 minutes or until chicken is fall-off-the-bone tender.
- Garnish with cilantro and serve with roasted vegetables or pan-fried sweet potatoes or plantains.

This recipe is a family favorite handed down from my wife's grandparents in Ecuador. It is a delicious one-pot meal that truly captures the rich flavors of Latin American cuisine. Eating Seco de Pollo is as close to a South American vacation as you can get without leaving your kitchen.

BEEF STIR-FRY

1 pound lean, grass-fed beef

2 pounds fresh or frozen vegetables

1 clove garlic

1 inch fresh ginger, peeled

½ tsp. red pepper flakes

1 tbsp. olive oil

- Grate garlic and ginger, and then add red pepper flakes.
- Slice meat, and then brown in skillet, using olive or coconut oil if needed. Set aside.
- Sauté vegetables in olive oil until tender-crisp.
- Add meat and sauce, cook until meat is to desired temperature.

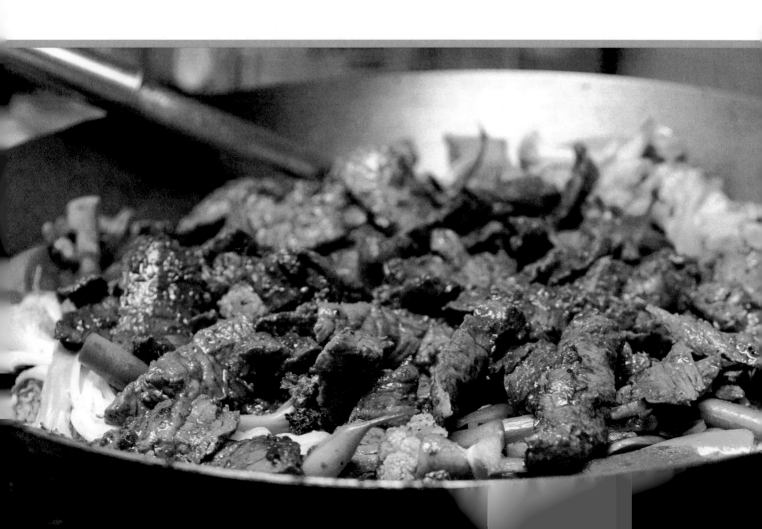

EGG FOO YUNG (ADAPTED FROM WELL FED)

2 whole omega-3 eggs plus 2 egg whites
4 oz. shredded or finely chopped chicken
2 cups shredded cabbage, sautéed or steamed until soft

1 tsp. Chinese five-spice powder*
¼ tsp. cayenne pepper or paprika
1 tbsp. olive oil
1 tsp. sesame oil
4 green onions sliced

- Whisk eggs and combine with other ingredients in mixing bowl.
- Heat large skillet to medium, add olive oil.
- Slowly pour egg mixture onto pan, forming a pancake about 3 or 4 inches across.
- Flip once eggs have set and pancake appears firm, about 5 minutes.
- Remove from heat once cooked evenly (10 minutes total).

*Chinese five-spice powder: equal parts cinnamon, cloves, ground fennel seed, star anise, and ground Szechuan peppercorns. (An easy cheat is to use cinnamon, ground cloves, and white pepper.)

DR. DAVE'S HEART-HEALTHY SOCAL FRIED CHICKEN

¼ cup olive oil
2 large omega-3 enriched eggs (or egg substitute)
1 cup almond flour
1 tsp. paprika

1 tsp. garlic powder
½ tsp. black pepper
2 pounds skinless chicken breasts, butterflied

- Heat oil in large frying pan on medium/high and preheat oven to 400°F.
- Whisk eggs in medium-sized bowl.
- Combine all dry ingredients in large bowl and mix well.
- Dip chicken in whisked eggs.
- Coat chicken with almond mixture and place in hot oil. Cook for about 2 minutes on each side, or until browned evenly.
- Place browned fillets on a baking sheet or pan and transfer to oven.
- Cook in oven for 10–15 minutes or until done.
- Remove and serve.

VEGGIES

I recommend that you keep a few bags of frozen vegetables in the house—broccoli, green beans, or mixed vegetable blends. You may find (as I do) that sometimes you have neither the time nor the energy to chop and wash vegetables. Especially when you are just getting started with your new lifestyle you will need some easy ways to get a serving of veggies on your plate. Frozen veggies can be defrosted in minutes and be ready on the table soon after. Pair sautéed or roasted vegetables with lean meats or tofu for a quick staple dinner.

Because you won't be having a big plate of rice or pasta with your dinner, be prepared to have lots more veggies ready than you might have been used to in the past. Don't be surprised if you end up serving up to one pound of vegetables per person at the table. Even though it sounds like a lot, an entire pound of green vegetables like broccoli or spinach has only about 100 calories.

"MASHED POTATOES"

1 head cauliflower, cut into florets   2-3 cloves garlic

- Add cauliflower and peeled garlic to steamer and cook until soft.
- Use a food processor to blend until smooth.

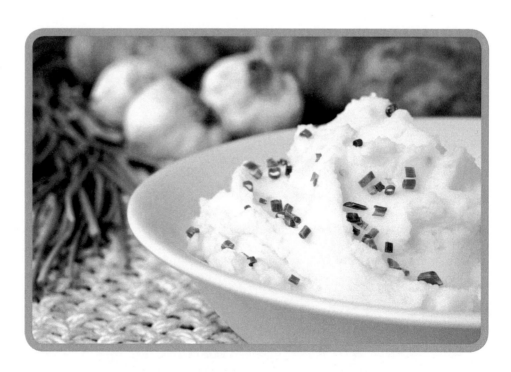

CAULIFLOWER FRIED "RICE"

1 head cauliflower, cut into florets

- In small batches run through food processor until the consistency is like rice.
- Cook in microwave for 2 min or stir-fry until desired texture.

KALE CHIPS

Kale   Salt-free seasoning blend

Olive oil

- Preheat oven to 275°F.
- Separate leaves from central stem and place in mixing bowl.
- Toss lightly with olive oil, salt-free seasoning blend, and pepper until coated.
- Spread evenly on cookie sheet and bake 10–15 min or until crunchy, rotating halfway through.
- Enjoy as soon as possible!

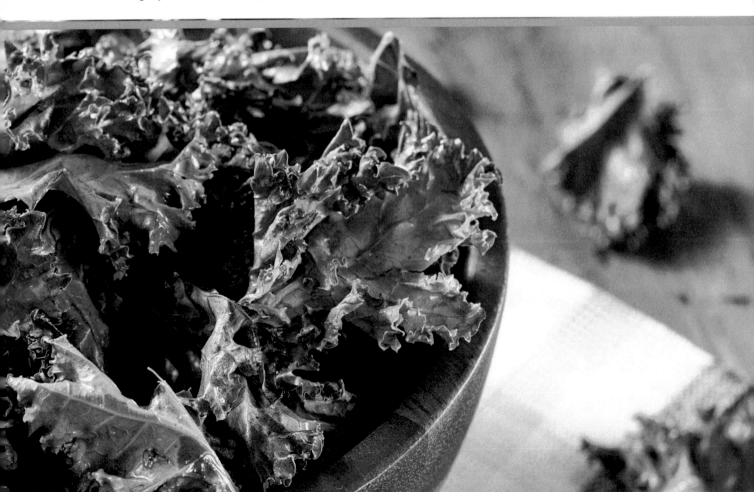

Most vegetables are excellent steamed, roasted, pan-fried, or stir-fried in some olive oil alone or with spices. Broccoli, cauliflower, asparagus, carrots, beets, and sweet potatoes are just a few examples. Experiment with different spices for variety.

ROASTED CARROTS

10 carrots
½ tbsp. cumin
¼ tsp. curry powder

¼ tsp. pepper
1½ tbsp. olive oil
Minced parsley

- Preheat oven to 400°F.
- Cut carrots lengthwise and then in half.
- Toss with olive oil and spices.
- Bake for 15–20 min on a foil-lined cookie sheet.

ROASTED BROCCOLI

2 pounds chopped broccoli florets
Olive oil

Garlic powder
Cayenne pepper

- Preheat oven to 400°F.
- Toss broccoli with olive oil and spices.
- Roast for about 15–20 or until tender.

ROASTED BEETS

Beets
Olive oil

Pepper

- Preheat oven 425°F.
- Peel beets, toss with olive oil and pepper.
- Spread on baking sheet covered in foil.
- Roast for 30 min. or until tender.

BRUSSELS SPROUTS AND SHALLOTS

1–2 pounds Brussels sprouts, quartered
2 shallots, thinly sliced

Olive oil
Pepper

- Preheat oven to 375°F.
- Toss Brussels sprouts and shallots with olive oil and pepper.
- Spread in one layer on a baking sheet covered in foil, bake until tender.

SAUTÉED CABBAGE AND APPLES

1 bag of shredded red cabbage
1 green apple, diced
1 small onion, sliced thin

Olive oil
2–4 tbsp. apple cider vinegar

- Sauté onions in olive oil.
- When soft, add cabbage.
- Cook cabbage until it starts to soften.
- Add the apple cider vinegar.
- Add apples and cook until apples are soft.

ROASTED EGGPLANT WITH GARLIC (ADAPTED FROM EMERIL LAGASSE)

1–2 large eggplants
4–5 cloves garlic

Olive oil

- Preheat oven to 400°F.
- Cut garlic lengthwise into small slivers.
- Slice 1–2 large eggplants into round wheels, ½ inch thick.
- Make little cuts in the eggplant wheels and insert slivers of garlic.
- Paint both sides with olive oil and arrange on baking sheet.
- Bake for about 20–25 minutes or until tender.

SIMPLE PALEO VEGGIE QUICHE (ADAPTED FROM KOHLERCREATED.COM)

7 omega-3 eggs
1½ cups chopped spinach
1 cup chopped broccoli
1 small onion chopped
3–4 cloves garlic, finely minced

½ cup coconut milk
Salt-free seasoning blend and/or black pepper to taste
Almond meal

- Preheat oven to 350°F.
- Whisk eggs and coconut milk, then blend with remaining ingredients.
- Grease a 9-inch pie tin with coconut oil, then coat evenly with almond meal.
- Add the egg mixture, then bake for about 40 minutes or until cooked evenly throughout.

LABOR OF LOVE EGGPLANT VEGGIE LASAGNA (ADAPTED FROM WELL FED)

3 medium eggplants
2 tbsp. olive oil
1 pound chopped/ground meat or chopped mushrooms
3 cloves garlic, minced

28 oz. jar of reduced sodium tomato sauce
8 large basil leaves
4 omega-3 eggs

- Preheat oven to 400°F.
- Slice eggplant ½ inch thick and place on baking sheets lined with parchment paper.
- Rub olive oil and ground pepper on both sides of eggplant and bake for 20 min.
- Reduce oven temperature to 350°F.
- While eggplant is roasting, brown the meat. Remove from pan and set aside.
- In the same pan, cook garlic until fragrant and then add the tomatoes and basil.
- Bring to a boil then reduce heat and simmer for 10 min. Let mixture cool.
- Scramble eggs in a bowl then add to the tomato mixture.

- Grease a 13x9 baking dish with olive oil. Layer eggplant, then meat, then tomato mixture.
- Repeat twice more, ending with tomato mixture on top.
- Bake for 30 min., remove and let rest for 30 min. before serving.

This eggplant lasagna recipe is one of my favorites, and as the name implies, it truly is a labor of love. Do not attempt unless you have plenty of time on your hands. But trust me, if you can make the time and put in the effort, you will get to enjoy an absolutely phenomenal dish. Hats off to the folks at Well Fed for coming up with this gem.

TIPS FOR YOUR MEAL PLAN

Here are a few last tips for making delicious, healthy meals without a lot of fuss or investment.

BREAKFAST

If you are busy, consider starting your day with a smoothie. A few ideas can be found among the recipes in this book. Also, breakfast foods reheat well, so making a few at a time is an efficient way to prepare ahead.

Staple breakfasts include egg scrambles, frittatas, one-minute muffins, and pancakes. Prepare them ahead of time and make a large batch. Save time and cook breakfast for the next day while you've got dinner in the oven.

Breakfast out should be scrambled eggs, fruits, vegetables, and lean meats or fish. Stay away from sandwich shops, and favor diners or restaurants. Thankfully in SoCal there is no shortage of Mexican eateries that will make a plate with eggs, vegetables, and chicken.

LUNCH

Lunches will often be leftovers from the night before (you have to sacrifice variety for convenience). Options for eating out include Mexican food (chicken or fish, beans, vegetables, salsa, and guacamole), salads, or simple entrees. Avoid sandwich shops, bakeries, and cafes. Never order anything with bread, tortillas, or rice, but ask for extra veggies instead. Most places will be happy to do so.

DINNER

If you don't have time for elaborate fare, grilled or roasted meats with copious amounts of vegetables are good, easy staple meals. Rotisserie chicken is always good in a pinch. When eating out order simply, avoiding sauces and substituting vegetables for potatoes or rice.

SNACKS

Nuts, fruits, and fresh vegetables are all good snacks. If you are at a desk or at home, have small meals more frequently so you have less need for snacking.

Good desserts include fresh fruits such as pears, apples, or berries with dark chocolate (at least 60% cocoa) in moderation.

That's it for the first Challenge. Keep a diet log, play with some recipes, and above all, have fun! When you've mastered the art of living like a caveman it's time to move on to the next Challenge. Good luck!

Steve M., age 52

I've been an underactive, overweight, middle-aged guy suffering from the all too common ailments typical of our fast-paced American lifestyle. I have tried many diets, many of which worked short-term before the yo-yo effect kicked in, because you can't live on bars or shakes for the rest of your life.

Meeting Dr. Dave and joining his program has put me on the long, hard, and incredibly rewarding road to extending my life and radically improving its quality. The results speak for themselves. When I met Dr. Dave, my hemoglobin A1c was 7.9, which meant that my average blood sugar was running around 180. I was on my way to more medication for my diabetes. Instead, I joined the program and only eight months later my average blood sugar is down to 117, my blood pressure is now way into the normal range, and I'm actually planning to start dropping medications!

What's important to me is that I am NOT on a diet; I am on a journey of lifestyle changes to take control of my physical health—with a physician who truly cares, understands, and stands by me every step of the way. We have a great group of guys in similar situations and we have bonded around our goals of improving our lives and battling these American lifestyle diseases. This program is not easy. It is not full of magic promises and mythical bars, shakes, or pills—but rather full of common sense, hard work, camaraderie, and results.

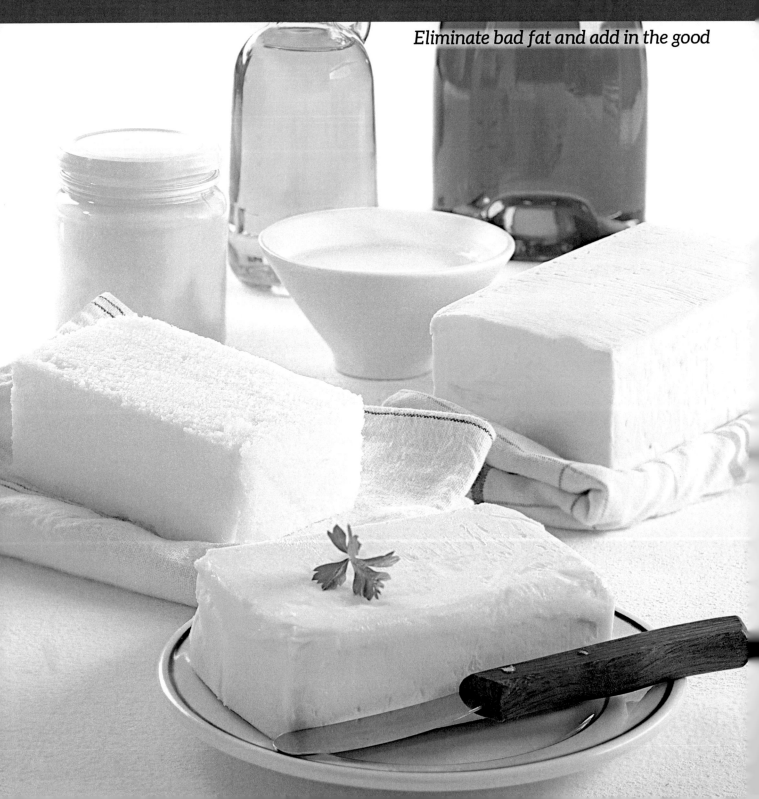

CHALLENGE #2: GET FAT!

Eliminate bad fat and add in the good

WHAT OUR ANCESTRAL DIET LACKS IN CARBOHYDRATES IT MAKES UP FOR IN FAT. This is not necessarily a bad thing—without the excess carbohydrates in the Western diet, you will need an alternate source of fuel. In fact, over one-third of the calories in the typical American diet come from carbohydrates in grains and added sugars. Take those away and you've got a lot of room on your plate to fill.

Exactly how you do that is an important question; the type of fat we ingest has the potential to radically alter our body's chemistry and consequently our health. Understanding and controlling this impact goes a long way to getting healthy and off medications.

WE'LL START WITH THE BASICS. WHAT IS FAT?

As much as I'd like to avoid it, we're going to have to start with some basic chemistry. Fats, fatty acids, or lipids are long chains of carbon surrounded by hydrogen atoms. Each carbon in the chain has four bonds; one each to the two adjacent carbons and one each to two hydrogen atoms. Only the last carbon is different, because it is bound to one carbon and to two oxygen atoms.

These chains of carbon and hydrogen are an excellent source of energy; a gram of fat contains about twice as many calories as a gram of sugar. When fats aren't being stored or burned they have other roles critical to our health. For example, the membrane surrounding every individual cell in your body is composed primarily of lipids. Also, many of the chemical messengers carrying signals throughout your body are specialized fat molecules.

There are three ways that fats differ based on their chemical structure. First there is the length of the chain. Fats range from short chains of as few as 4-5 carbon atoms, to medium chains of up to 12 carbon atoms, and long chains of as many as 20 or more carbon atoms.

Next is the degree of saturation of the fat molecule. If a carbon is joined to its neighboring carbon atom by a single chemical bond then each can also bond with two hydrogen atoms. This configuration is called saturated because the carbon atoms are completely saturated with hydrogen.

Saturated Fat

If the carbon atoms are joined by a double bond, each carbon can bond only one, not two, hydrogen atoms. In this case the molecule is called unsaturated. Every double bond is a point of unsaturation. A fat with one double bond is monounsaturated; a fat with two or more double bonds is polyunsaturated.

Monosaturated Fat

The last difference among fats is the location of each of the double bonds. Unsaturated fats are named for the location of the first double bond; for example, the omega-3 fats have the first double bond three carbons away from the oxygen atom at one end of the molecule.

Polyunsaturated Fat

Notice that a molecule of saturated fat is straight while the unsaturated fats are kinked. The flat configuration of saturated fats allows them to pack together tighter than poly- or monounsaturated fats. This affects their melting point; saturated fats tend to be solid at room temperature while unsaturated fats are liquid. Any fat that you can cut with a knife, such as butter or coconut oil, is likely to be saturated fat. The only exception to this rule of thumb is the much-maligned trans-fat.

Trans-fats are man-made fats created by adding extra hydrogen to a polyunsaturated fat to make it act more like a saturated fat. The idea originally was to make a polyunsaturated fat that was solid at room temperature and cheap enough to use for mass food production. Unfortunately, we kind of dropped the ball on this one; it turns out that trans-fats are the worst kinds of fats for clogging up arteries. Trans-fats are slowly being removed from the food supply although they still turn up at restaurants and in processed foods, including a few unlikely places like non-dairy creamer. Avoid fried foods at restaurants and stay true to your hunter-gatherer roots so that you won't cross paths with these true modern villains.

THERE'S STRENGTH IN NUMBERS

Fatty acids are rarely found floating around all by themselves; instead they are usually stored and transported in the form of triglycerides. A triglyceride is composed of three fatty acids linked together by a molecule of glycerol.

Triglyceride molecule
(composed of three saturated fatty acids bound together by glycerol)

Most of the fat we ingest is in the form of triglycerides. We can't absorb triglycerides directly; bile acids secreted by the gallbladder and enzymes secreted by the pancreas break down ingested triglycerides into individual fatty acids. These fatty acids are then absorbed and reassembled into triglycerides for transportation and storage inside our body. When we talk about fats we are usually talking about triglycerides.

YOU CAN'T STOMACH FAT WITHOUT CHOLESTEROL

Cholesterol is what makes the digestion of fat possible. Cholesterol has a number of important roles in our body: it is an integral part of the lipid membrane surrounding every cell and is the basis for hormones such as testosterone, estrogen, and even vitamin D. Cholesterol is also the backbone of bile salts, which are critical to our ability to digest fat. In fact, most of the cholesterol made by the liver each day is sent to the gallbladder for this very purpose. Cholesterol is used to manufacture bile salts, which are then stored in the gallbladder and released into our intestines after a fatty meal. The bile salts mix with the fat in our diet and break up triglycerides into individual fatty acids to be absorbed.

Bile salts and cholesterol we ingest from food sources are partially absorbed in the intestines and travel to the liver to be processed. About one-third of our daily cholesterol comes from intestinal absorption and the other two thirds is manufactured each day in the liver. Other animals make cholesterol too—in fact, cholesterol is only found in animal products; animal fat, to be specific. Plants do not make cholesterol, but do make similar molecules called sterols that are discussed in the section on supplements.

When we measure cholesterol we don't measure the concentration of actual cholesterol, but rather the concentration of transport proteins that carry cholesterol throughout the body. The metrics that appear on most cholesterol tests include total cholesterol, LDL (low-density lipoprotein), HDL (high-density lipoprotein), IDL (intermediate-density lipoprotein), VLDL (very-low-density lipoprotein), and triglycerides. Lipoprotein is the name for any protein-based molecule that is used to transport fat and cholesterol throughout the body.

You'll notice that the proteins are named for their density. Each lipoprotein is analogous to a bus that is designed to carry fat and cholesterol throughout the body to various destinations. Since fat is less dense than water, lipoproteins that carry more fat are less dense. VLDL is the least dense because it carries the most fat, while HDL is the densest because it carries the least amount of fat.

Lipoproteins are made in the liver and start their journey there. They travel from the liver throughout the body, carrying fat and cholesterol to wherever they are needed. Each cell in the body can express receptors for LDL and other lipoproteins, making each organ the equivalent of a bus stop that can be open or closed to receiving passengers.

As the lipoproteins drop off fat they become denser. As they become denser they change form, evolving from VLDL to IDL and LDL. All of these lipoproteins are responsible for carrying fat and cholesterol *away* from the liver, which is why they are all commonly grouped together as "bad" cholesterol. Triglycerides, measured separately, are another form of bad cholesterol.

HDL is the "good" lipoprotein that carries cholesterol in the opposite direction, from the body back to the liver. Once HDL makes it back to the liver, it drops off its cholesterol for conversion into bile salts that are then excreted. Although there are many forms of bad cholesterol, HDL is the only form of good cholesterol.

WHEN GOOD ARTERIES GO BAD

The process of going from nice clean arteries to a heart attack or stroke takes decades and starts with an accumulation of LDL (bad cholesterol) in the bloodstream. When LDL levels creep up past a certain threshold, the lipids contained in the LDL particle become susceptible to oxidation. Oxidized lipids are free radicals that damage surrounding molecules and disrupt the normal functioning of the body. Oxidation occurs when fats (or other molecules) are exposed to energy (usually heat or light) in the presence of oxygen. Cooking, especially at high heats, causes oxidation of fats; however, fats can also become oxidized after they've been ingested and become part of an LDL particle. Physical or emotional stress, smoking, lack of sleep, and other factors can increase the amount of oxidation that occurs in the body. We'll discuss oxidation in more detail during Challenge #5 when we work on antioxidants.

Our first line of defense against oxidized LDL is to take it out of the bloodstream before it can cause any damage. Our immune system targets oxidized LDL particles by sending certain immune cells called macrophages to gobble them up like Pac-Man. After eating its fill of oxidized LDL, a macrophage becomes what is called a "foam cell." These foam cells, along with their load of cholesterol and oxidized fat, eventually come to rest along the walls of your arteries.

Once the foam cell settles in the wall of the artery, your body sets up a second line of defense. Over time a thick layer of fibrous tissue covers the foam cells and becomes calcified like bone. These calcified plaques in the walls of the artery are a hallmark of advanced vascular disease, and can be seen on CT scans and even X-rays of the chest and other body parts.

If that were the end of the story then there wouldn't be much worry about vascular disease. Oxidized LDL would get walled off and we'd forget about it. Unfortunately, there's more. The calcified plaque may remain dormant, in which case there really may be no problem. But in some cases the immune system continues to target the plaque, causing it to become inflamed—much the same way picking at a small pimple turns it into a big angry sore. The hard surface of the plaque erodes and eventually ruptures, spilling foam cells and calcium plaque into the artery. Blood cells called "platelets" clump around the broken plaque and form a clot that blocks the artery completely, killing any organ that is downstream. If that organ is your brain, we call it a stroke; if it is your heart, we call it a heart attack. Either way it is bad news.

WHAT'S DIET GOT TO DO WITH IT?

Let's take a look at how dietary fat and cholesterol play a role in each step of the process, starting with the high LDL levels. What drives up LDL in the first place? You might think that eating more cholesterol is to blame, and you'd be partly right. The liver makes about 800 milligrams of cholesterol per day, compared to about 300 milligrams in a typical balanced diet. Because diet only contributes a third of the total day's cholesterol, even relatively big swings in dietary cholesterol may change your blood levels by only about 10–15%.

Dietary cholesterol is but one part of the equation. Another big determinant of blood cholesterol levels is the amount and type of fat in our diet. Earlier we talked about how each cell in our body has receptors for LDL cholesterol. Expression of these receptors on the surface of the cell is regulated by genes, which in turn are regulated in part by the amount of saturated fat in the diet. A diet high in saturated fat down-regulates LDL receptor genes, reducing the number of receptors and increasing blood levels of LDL. Decreasing saturated fat in the diet up-regulates these genes, creating more receptors for LDL on the surface of cells. These receptors then pull more LDL out of circulation to be put to good use. This is why doctors often recommend reducing the amount of saturated fat in the diet.

Monounsaturated and polyunsaturated fats have the opposite effect of saturated fats and actually reduce the amount of LDL in circulation. Therefore, swapping out saturated fat for monounsaturated fats and polyunsaturated fats lowers LDL cholesterol.

---

*Saturated fat increases LDL. Monounsaturated
and polyunsaturated fats decrease LDL.*

Oxidation of the LDL is the second step in the progression of heart disease. Here's where the story gets complicated. Oxidation of a fat molecule can occur only if the fat molecule has a double bond. Fats with more double bonds (e.g., polyunsaturated fats) are more likely to be oxidized when exposed to stress, light, or heat. Polyunsaturated fats are very prone to oxidation, while saturated fats are resistant to oxidation. Monounsaturated fats, which have only one double bond, also resist oxidation.

Thus, while saturated fats such as those found in coconut oil or butter may increase the amount of LDL, they also are the most resistant to oxidation and consequently may be less likely to end up in the walls of your arteries inside foam cells. The jury is still out on what this means for saturated fats and health—are they good because they don't oxidize or are they bad because they increase LDL to begin with? The answer isn't straightforward and will probably be debated for some time to come.

Monounsaturated fats such as those found in olive oil, nuts, and avocados also resist oxidation and, unlike saturated fats, reduce LDL. In contrast to the controversy surrounding saturated fats, it is pretty much universally accepted that decreasing LDL and resisting oxidation at the same time is very good for you. Throw in the fact that olives and olive oil are also packed with antioxidants and you can see why the Mediterranean diet is so effective in preventing heart disease.

---

*Saturated fats and monounsaturated fats resist oxidation.
Polyunsaturated fats oxidize easily.*

The last step in the progression of heart disease is inflammation of the cholesterol plaque. This step is mediated by the amount and type of polyunsaturated fat in our diet. The two polyunsaturated fats that regulate inflammation are the omega-3 and omega-6 fats, named for the location of the first double bond (the third and sixth carbon atoms, respectively). The balance of omega-3 and omega-6 in our diet is responsible for the inflammation of the cholesterol plaque as well as other inflammatory disorders, including arthritis and asthma.

Inflammation in the body is dependent on the amount of omega-6 fatty acids in the diet. **Linoleic acid (LA)** is the primary omega-6 in the diet and is metabolized in the body to **arachidonic acid**. Arachidonic acid is a chemical mediator that increases inflammation and platelet aggregation (promotes clot formation). Both steps are critical to the development of heart attack and stroke. Arachidonic acid is so important to these conditions that we give our patients at risk of heart disease medication to block its action. This medication is aspirin, and if you are taking a baby aspirin a day, you are taking this medication to offset the effect of omega-6 in your diet. Other medications that block the action of arachidonic acid include ibuprofen (Advil or Motrin), naproxen (Aleve), and prednisone, a prescription medication commonly prescribed for everything from arthritis to asthma.

Omega-3 fatty acids have the exact opposite role from omega-6 fatty acids. Omega-3 fats are the "good" polyunsaturated fatty acids that reduce inflammation in the body and block the chemical signaling that causes blood clots, thereby reducing the risk of heart disease and stroke. **Alpha-linolenic acid (ALA)** is an omega-3 fatty acid that is then converted in our body to **docosohexaenoic acid (DHA)** and **eicosapentaenoic acid (EPA)**. DHA and EPA are then metabolized into **prostaglandins**, which are chemical mediators that inhibit inflammation and improve platelet function. More omega-3s in the diet means more prostaglandins and less inflammation. Omega-3s also affect cholesterol metabolism, reducing triglycerides and modestly increasing HDL (good cholesterol).

Omega-3s also have wide-ranging benefits outside the circulatory system. Studies have shown that omega-3 fats can reduce the symptoms of inflammatory arthritis and supplementation in childhood can prevent and treat asthma. Perhaps most importantly, omega-3s are an important contributor to brain cell functioning. Dietary DHA is critical in infancy to the development of a healthy brain and nervous system. In adulthood, DHA and omega-3s have been linked to the prevention of Alzheimer's disease. The list of benefits seems endless.

Omega-3 ALA is found in certain plants like walnuts, chia, and flax, as well as in small amounts in green vegetables and grasses. DHA and EPA are found in grass-fed meat, dairy from grass-fed cows, fish, and algae. Omega-6 fats are found in grains, corn, soybeans, and most nuts, as well as most dairy and store-bought meats. As we read earlier, commercial farms use grain-based feeds that are high in omega-6. These omega-6 fats make it into the meat, eggs, and milk that end up on your plate.

A balanced caveman diet would have an approximate 2:1 ratio of omega-6 to omega-3 fats. This is the optimal ratio to maintain a healthy but not excessive, level of inflammation in your body.

Omega-6 fats increase inflammation while omega-3 fats decrease it. The ideal ratio of omega-6 to omega-3 in the diet is 2:1.

In contrast to our caveman diet, an American diet, even a healthy one, has about ten times more omega-6 than omega-3. All the grains, corn, and grain-fed meat are laden with omega-6 and devoid of omega-3. With a balance like this, is it any wonder that heart disease and other inflammatory diseases are so common?

Omega-6 fatty acids, obesity, and natural selection.

Never before in the history of mankind have we had so little omega-3 and so much omega-6. It is not by coincidence that this dramatic shift in our diet happens to coincide with a dramatic increase in worldwide obesity rates. Studies suggest that omega-6 fats directly promote obesity by directing the body to preferentially store fats around the abdomen and internal organs. Furthermore, the obesity epidemic caused by the introduction of omega-6 and processed carbohydrates to our environment may be the latest stage in the evolution of man.

Animal studies show that a diet rich in omega-6 fatty acids, even when total calories are held constant, leads to preferential storage of fat around the abdomen. Excess calories from fat or carbohydrates only exacerbate the problem. Fat accumulates around the internal organs, leading to diabetes and a host of other problems.

It isn't just the excess calories that cause obesity; the omega-6 fats cause cells to express otherwise dormant genes that direct the body to store fat in the abdomen, where it does the most harm. These changes to gene expression are called "epigenetic changes." Epigenetic changes are hereditary and get passed down from generation to generation. Animal studies confirm that children of parents who were fed a high omega-6 diet are born with these genes expressed and are predisposed to obesity right from the womb. When these children are also fed a high-omega-6 diet the cycle builds on itself with each successive generation.

These epigenetic changes, if applicable to humans, would predict a rise in childhood obesity, and of course that is exactly what is happening today. When we gorge on omega-6 fats before we reach childbearing age, not only do we get fat but our kids are more likely to be obese. Their genes are programmed to store fat around the midsection right from birth. As these children consume the same diet as their parents did, a death spiral occurs with each subsequent generation becoming more obese earlier in life.

Now for the scary part: human studies show that obesity leads to a significant reduction in fertility for both men and women. Compared with their thinner contemporaries, men and women who are overweight are less likely to have a successful pregnancy and healthy child. Does this sound like anything you've read about in the earlier sections of this book? It should. Given enough time, natural selection tells us that only those lucky few who are genetically immune to the effects of omega-6 (or those smart enough to avoid them) will populate the Earth. A sobering thought, to be sure, and only the next 100,000 years will tell us if this is indeed the case.

Before you kiss the human race goodbye, there is a glimmer of hope. Thankfully, animal studies show that this epigenetic programming is completely reversible. Animals that were born to obese parents start out obese, but if their diet is changed back to one rich in omega-3, the genes are turned off and the obesity is reversed. So before you chalk up any health problems to "genetics," remember that very little is actually outside your control.

THE SKINNY ON FATS

Here's the bottom line. Saturated fats raise LDL cholesterol but resist oxidation. Monounsaturated fats lower LDL and also resist oxidation. Polyunsaturated fats lower LDL but are easily oxidized. Omega-6 polyunsaturated fats cause inflammation and obesity while omega-3 fats reduce inflammation and may prevent obesity. To put it in simple terms of good and bad:

- *Omega-3s are good*
- *Omega-6s are bad*
- *Monounsaturated fats are good*
- *Saturated fats might be good or bad*

SATURATED FAT; FRIEND OR FOE?

The question of whether saturated fat is good or bad is still unanswered, although there is a strong argument to be made that perhaps saturated fats aren't the villains we once thought they were. The main dietary sources of saturated fats are meats and animal fat, dairy, coconuts, and palm. As we've read earlier, there is a significant body of evidence that meat is associated with an increased risk of heart disease. This may be due to the saturated fat; however, it might also be due to other factors such as carnitine and choline or to the oxidation of polyunsaturated fats during cooking. Either could possibly explain the link between meat and heart disease.

This would suggest that eliminating saturated fat from all sources might be unnecessary, as it might not be the saturated fat in meat that causes heart disease but these other factors instead. If so, then enjoying saturated fat from other (i.e., plant and dairy) sources might be safe and may even reduce the risk of heart disease.

Some studies do show that certain populations with extreme diets such as Eskimos (all fish and blubber) or tropical villagers (all coconuts and palm) actually have less heart disease than we have here in the U.S. The question is whether this would apply to us. One thing to remember is that our prehistoric ancestors did not have refined oils; these are a recent addition to the human diet. Eskimos and tropical villagers get their food whole. There's a big difference between eating a whole coconut and buying a jar of coconut oil that can be ladled out by the spoonful. Loading up on coconut oil or any other source of saturated fat is likely to raise your LDL well beyond the levels seen in any population with a low incidence of heart disease.

It is doubtful that the question of a "safe" level of saturated fats will be settled anytime soon. Trials evaluating the links between diet and disease are difficult to plan and even more difficult to execute. A balanced diet contains innumerable foods that vary over time and often obfuscate any possible links between one factor (e.g., saturated fat) and the incidence of disease. It is therefore unlikely that the debate on saturated fats will be resolved in the foreseeable future.

In the meantime, the safest strategy is to emphasize monounsaturated and omega-3 fats in the diet, and enjoy coconut and other saturated fats only in moderation.

TURNING KNOWLEDGE INTO ACTION

Now that we've learned more than you ever wanted to know about fats, it's time to turn our attention to the kitchen. We're going to want to emphasize monounsaturated fats and omega-3s as much as possible, and limit the amount of omega-6 and saturated fat. Here are some specific tips for putting your knowledge into action.

#1 Avoid processed foods

Eliminating saturated fat and omega-6 starts with our caveman diet. Modern processed foods are usually packed with both saturated and omega-6 fat. Cookies, crackers, bars, chips, even breads and pastries all usually contain both types of unhealthy fat; for example, a bagel contains about 3.5 grams of saturated and omega-6 fat. Avoiding anything that comes in a bag or a box will help you weed these out of your diet.

#2 Buy pasture-raised meats and keep to leaner cuts

Grain-fed meat has about a 10:1 ratio or more of omega-6 to omega-3. Lose the store-bought meat and you'll reduce the amount of omega-6 in your diet. If you were enjoying fatty cuts of meat (including bacon or other processed meats) during the first Challenge, now is the time to rein it in. Start opting for leaner cuts, make sure the meat is pasture-raised, and avoid any excess fat.

#3 Cook with olive, avocado, or coconut oils. Canola oil only cold and in moderation.

When choosing cooking oil, the most important consideration is the amount of oxidation. Cooking naturally involves heat and oxygen, just the recipe for free radicals. For this reason it makes sense to limit our choices to the oils with the highest amount of monounsaturated and saturated fats, both of which resist oxidation. We want to avoid even healthy omega-3 fats during cooking since they, like all polyunsaturated fats, will oxidize when heated.

The next consideration is the impact on our cholesterol levels. Olive and avocado oils are highest in the monounsaturated fats that lower LDL and raise HDL. These should therefore be preferred over other oils.

If we are going to use an oil cold then we can tolerate polyunsaturated fat as long as there is the right ratio of omega-6 to omega-3. I would not use safflower oil for cooking because, even though it has about the same amount of monounsaturated fat as olive or avocado oils, it has much more omega-6. On the other hand, canola oil has the perfect 2:1 ratio of omega-6 to omega-3 that we are looking for, so it could be used for cold applications like salad dressings. Canola oil is difficult to recommend only because it must be processed in order to remove toxins found in the rapeseed plant from which the oil is derived. Processing is technically a no-no, but the reality is that having some canola oil in the diet is unlikely to make or break you. I'll let you decide whether or not you need it in your diet.

Fatty acid composition of common vegetable oils

	FAT (g)					
	SF	MUFA	PUFA	n-6	n-3	n-6:n-3
Butter	7.2	2.9	0.4	0.3	0.0	7:1
Olive	1.9	10.2	1.5	1.4	0.1	13:1
Avocado	1.6	9.9	1.9	1.8	0.1	13:1
Canola	1.0	8.9	3.9	2.6	1.3	2:1
Safflower	1.1	10.5	1.8	1.8	0.0	> 100:1
Sunflower	1.4	2.7	9.2	9.2	0.0	> 100:1
Palm	6.9	5.2	1.3	1.3	0.0	46:1
Soybean	2.2	3.2	8.1	7.1	1.0	8:1
Corn	1.8	3.9	7.7	7.5	0.2	46:1
Coconut	12.1	0.8	0.3	0.0	0.3	0:1
Walnut	1.3	3.2	8.9	7.4	1.5	5:1

per tablespoon (14 grams)

SF: saturated fat, MUFA: monounsaturated fat, PUFA: polyunsaturated fat, n-6: omega-6, n-3: omega-3

#4 Enjoy nuts, focusing on walnuts, almonds, pistachios, cashews, and macadamia nuts

Although nuts tend to be high in omega-6, they are still an important part of a healthy, all-natural diet. Nuts are one of the few foods that have consistently been shown to reduce the risk of heart disease and cardiac death. They are also packed with vitamins, minerals, fiber, and sterols, which are all important to your health. Plant sterols in particular are useful for lowering cholesterol and may account for some of their benefit. Read ahead to the appendix to learn more about sterols and health. Of the popular tree nuts, cashews, macadamia nuts, pistachios, and almonds have the least omega-6. Walnuts have the most polyunsaturated fat and omega-6 but have a better omega-6 to omega-3 ratio than most other nuts.

		FAT (g)				
	SF	MUFA	PUFA	n-6	n-3	n-6:n-3
Almond	1.5	12.4	4.8	4.8	0.0	> 100:1
Walnut	2.4	3.6	18.8	15.2	3.6	4:1
Peanut	2.7	9.8	6.2	6.2	0.0	> 100:1
Pecan	2.5	16.3	8.6	8.2	0.4	21:1
Cashew	3.1	9.5	3.1	3.1	0.0	> 100:1
Pistachio	2.2	9.5	5.5	5.4	0.1	68:1
Macadamia	4.8	23.5	0.6	0.5	0.1	7:1

per 40 g raw portion (about one handful)

#5 Emphasize fish, chia, and flax for omega-3s

Fish, chia, and flax are the most concentrated sources of omega-3 fat in the diet. The best sources of omega-3 are listed in the table below, along with more details on their fat profiles than you probably want to know. A quarter pound serving of herring, sardine, salmon, tuna, or anchovy is enough to supply your daily omega-3 requirement.

	FAT (g)				n-3 (grams)			
	SF	MUFA	PUFA	n-6	ALA	EPA+DHA[1]	Total n-3	n-6:n-3
Herring	2.0	3.7	2.1	0.1	0.1	1.6	1.7	0.1
Flaxseed (ground)	0.3	0.5	2.0	0.4	1.6	0.0	1.6	0.3
Sardine (canned in oil)	1.5	3.9	5.1	3.5	0.5	1.0	1.5	2.4
Anchovy	1.3	1.2	1.6	0.1	0.0	1.5	1.5	0.1
Tuna (bluefin)	1.3	1.6	1.4	0.1	0.0	1.3	1.3	0.0
Salmon	1.2	1.9	1.7	0.4	1.3	0.0	1.3	0.3
Chia	0.2	0.2	1.7	0.4	1.3	0.0	1.3	0.3
Trout	0.7	1.1	1.2	0.2	0.1	0.7	0.8	0.3
Catfish	0.7	0.8	0.9	0.3	0.1	0.5	0.5	0.5
Halibut	0.3	0.5	0.3	0.0	0.0	0.2	0.2	0.1
Grass-fed beef (loin)	2.7	2.4	0.4	0.2	0.1	0.1	0.1	2.2
Grass-fed beef (ground, 85% lean)	7.9	0.8	0.7	0.3	0.1	0.0	0.1	2.2

per 100 grams

1. Includes contribution from DPA, which is an intermediary EPA and DHA

Notice that even though grass-fed beef has a near-perfect ratio of omega-6 to omega-3, it actually provides very little polyunsaturated fat and practically no omega-3; most of the omega-6 and omega-3 is turned into CLA during rumination. CLA is the cancer-fighting version of omega-3 and omega-6 that we covered earlier in the discussion about grass-fed beef and its many attributes. The conversion of omegas into CLA is one of the most potent selling points of grass-fed beef.

#6 Rely on chia and flax for omega-3 only if you're staying true to your caveman diet

Recall from our earlier discussion that plants contain omega-3 in the form of ALA, which we then metabolize into biologically active DHA and EPA before it can be used to fight inflammation. The same enzyme metabolizes both ALA (omega-3) and LA (omega-6). When the diet heavily favors omega-6 the enzymes responsible for converting plant omega-3 into EPA and DHA get backed up processing all that omega-6. If you are still indulging in store-bought meats, cheeses, or breads rich in omega-6, you are unlikely to see any benefit from throwing in some extra flaxseed or chia.

On the other hand, once you have a proper 2:1 balance of dietary omega-6 to omega-3 you are much more likely to be able to make good use of plant omega-3s. If there is any doubt that you've been cutting back on the omega-6 (for example, if you eat out often), you should plan to get your omega-3 as DHA and EPA from animal sources or algae.

HOW ABOUT CANNED TUNA FOR OMEGA-3S?

Canned tuna or salmon should never be preferred over the fresh variety; however, should you choose to go with a canned version, here are a few things to keep in mind. First of all, canned products may be very high in sodium, which we will cover in detail in another Challenge. Try to avoid high sodium products at all costs. Second, always choose a water-packed over an oil-packed fish. Fish packed in oil has more omega-6 than omega-3, which totally negates the whole point of eating fish in the first place. As you can see in the above table, sardines canned in oil are the only fish listed that have more omega-6 than omega-3.

HOW MUCH OMEGA-3 SHOULD I GET EACH DAY?

Many health authorities recommend a minimum intake of 1.2 grams omega-3 per day for women and 1.6 grams for men. Higher amounts, in the range of 2–3 grams per day, are effective for lowering triglycerides and increasing your good HDL cholesterol. I would suggest shooting for these more aggressive levels for maximum benefit. If you are falling short then be sure to fill in the gaps with a supplement that supplies both DHA and EPA.

YOUR MISSION, SHOULD YOU CHOOSE TO ACCEPT IT...

In this next Challenge we are going to put our hunter-gatherer skills to the test. We'll hunt for and eliminate the saturated fat and unhealthy omega-6 polyunsaturated fat in our diet, substituting instead healthy fats that will lower cholesterol, increase good cholesterol, and reduce (rather than increase) the risk of heart disease.

Monounsaturated fats in olive oil, avocados, and nuts have proven cardiovascular benefits. Now is the time to start enjoying them to your heart's content. Here in SoCal we are lucky to have year-round access to avocados. Take advantage of this and find some new ways to enjoy them.

Omega-3s are perhaps the most challenging to include in our diet so this is where you may need to put in the most effort during this Challenge. Flax, chia, omega-3 enriched eggs, and fish are powerful inflammation-fighting foods. Start including more varieties of fish and enjoy them more often. Learn some new recipes with plant-based omega-3 from flax and chia, starting with the *ridiculously* good Omega-Madness Muffin.

Challenge #2: Without deviating from your hunter-gatherer diet, identify all sources of saturated and omega-6 fats and replace them with monounsaturated fats and omega-3s. Include at least one serving per day of a plant-based omega-3 and get at least one serving of omega-3 from fish. You should aim for at least 2,000 milligrams of omega-3 each day.

BREAKFAST

FLAXSEED ALMOND MUFFINS

½ cup almond flour
½ cup flax meal
1 tsp. cinnamon
½ tsp. nutmeg
4 dates
4 omega-3 eggs

2 tbsp. olive oil
⅔ cup water
¼ cup finely chopped walnuts
½ cup shredded, unsweetened coconut
¼ cup dried or fresh chopped apples

- Preheat oven to 350°F.
- In a large bowl combine almond flour, flax meal, cinnamon, and nutmeg.
- In a blender, puree dates, apples, eggs, oil, and water on high speed until very smooth.
- Combine wet and dry ingredients in bowl, then stir in remaining ingredients.
- Spoon batter into greased muffin tins.
- Bake for 25–30 minutes (for six large muffins) or 17–22 minutes (for nine medium muffins). Muffins are done when a wooden stick comes out clean.
- Cool and serve.

Fish for breakfast? Crazy! Try these recipes for getting your DHA and EPA first thing in the morning. Also, remember when shopping for eggs to always get the omega-3 enriched ones. If you don't want the expense of omega-3 eggs just use plain egg whites, but avoid unenriched egg yolks if you can help it.

DR. DAVE'S OMEGA-3 MADNESS MUFFIN

3 tbsp. ground flaxseed
1 tsp. olive oil
1 omega-3 egg, lightly beaten
1 small ripe banana, mashed

½ tsp. vanilla extract
Cocoa powder, fresh berries, nuts or other additions as desired

- Combine ingredients and spoon into mug.
- Add any flavorings you like: chopped fruit, cinnamon, cocoa, or coconut.
- Microwave on high 2 minutes or longer depending on mug and microwave.
- Flip upside down to dislodge muffin. When ready it will be firm in the middle and have the consistency of thick oatmeal.

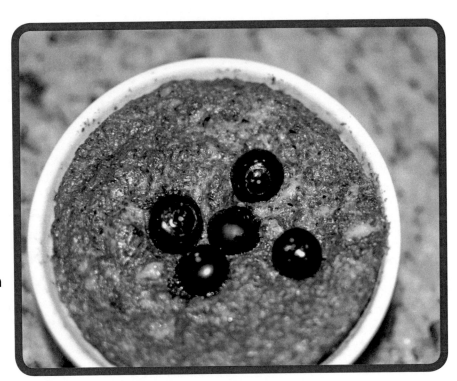

SCRAMBLED EGGS WITH FRESH ANCHOVIES

2 omega-3 eggs
1 tomato cut into wedges
½ onion, diced
2 cloves garlic, chopped
1 can whole peeled tomatoes

1 tbsp. paprika
1 tsp. oregano
4 fresh anchovy fillets, chopped finely
Olive oil

- Heat a pan with olive oil and sauté onions and garlic.
- Add tomatoes, followed by paprika and oregano.
- Bring to a simmer and add anchovies.

- Spread mixture evenly in pan, then with a spoon form two wells in the puree.
- Drop both eggs into the wells and cover pan, reducing heat to low.
- Cook until egg is done to your liking.
- Can be served with cooked sweet potatoes or other vegetables.

Canned fish, including sardines and anchovies, are heavily salted. Enjoy this recipe with fresh anchovy fillets and avoid the added sodium.

SALMON SALAD

2 cups cooked salmon fillet
2 omega-3 eggs, hard-boiled and crushed
1 green or red pepper, diced
1 cucumber, seeded and diced

¼ cup chopped onions
4 tbsp. olive oil
Dash of cayenne pepper
White or black pepper to taste
Juice of ½ lemon

- In a large mixing bowl, combine vegetables, seasonings, and olive oil and toss to mix thoroughly.
- Add salmon and eggs. Gently mix to combine.
- Drizzle with lemon juice. Serve.

LUNCH & DINNER

There are plenty of elaborate fish recipes out there, but we need some easy staple recipes for the everyday. Examples include broiled salmon or other fish; just brush the salmon with olive oil and dust with garlic and pepper then broil for about 10 minutes. But if you have the luxury of time and the creativity to try some new dishes, read on...

. . . .

ALMOND-CRUSTED SALMON FILLET

¾ pound salmon fillets
½ cup almond flour
½ tsp. ground coriander
½ tsp. ground cumin

Juice of 1 lemon
Freshly ground black pepper
Fresh cilantro
1 tbsp. coconut oil

- Preheat the oven to 350°F.
- Combine almond flour, coriander, and cumin in a small bowl.
- Sprinkle the salmon fillets with the lemon juice and season with pepper.
- Coat each fillet with the almond mixture.
- Place skin side down on a broiler pan, greased lightly with coconut oil.
- Bake for 12–15 minutes or until salmon flakes easily with a fork.
- Top with freshly chopped cilantro before serving.

. . . .

FENNEL SCENTED SALMON

1–2 salmon fillets
1 tsp. fennel seeds, crushed

¼ tsp. pepper
Olive oil

- Mix pepper and crushed fennel seeds together and coat salmon.
- Heat a pan with olive oil and cook salmon until done.

GINGER TUNA STEAKS

2 wild-caught tuna steaks

1" fresh ginger, sliced

1 tbsp. olive oil

- Combine ginger and olive oil in a gallon plastic bag.
- Add tuna steaks.
- Marinate tuna steaks for at least an hour.
- Grill.

SARDINE SALAD

3 tbsp. lemon juice

2 tbsp. extra virgin olive oil

1 clove garlic, minced

2 tsp. dried oregano

½ tsp. freshly ground pepper

3 medium tomatoes cut into large chunks

1 large English cucumber, cut into large chunks

1 15 oz. can chickpeas, rinsed

¼ cup thinly sliced red onion

2 tbsp. sliced olives

8 oz. sardines (If using fresh sardines, sauté them in olive oil prior to serving.)

- Whisk lemon juice, oil, garlic, oregano, and pepper in a large bowl until well combined.
- Add tomatoes, cucumber, chickpeas, feta, onion, and olives; gently toss to combine. Divide the salad among 4 plates and top with sardines.

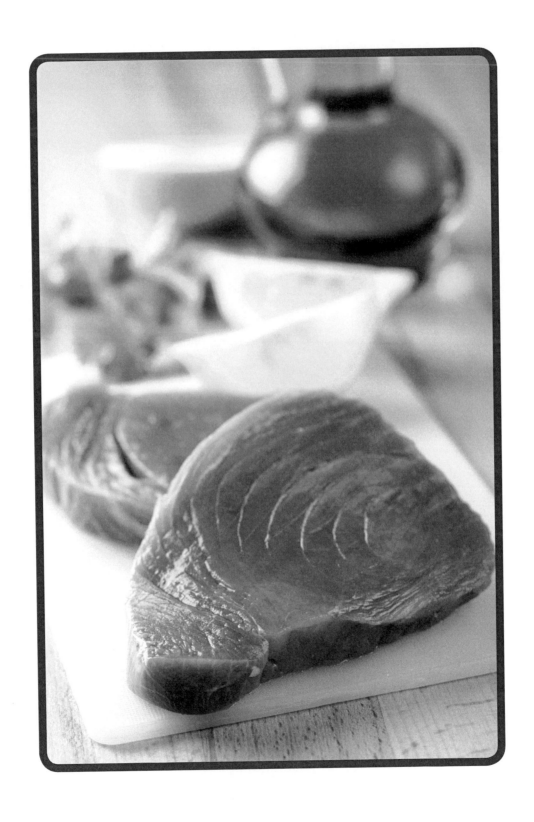

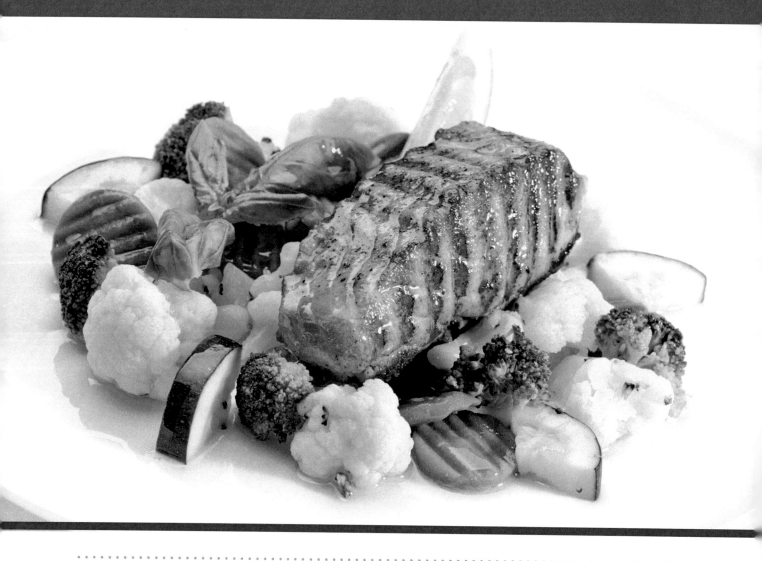

SPICED SALMON

1–2 pounds salmon

1 tbsp. olive oil

1 tbsp. orange juice

1½ tsp. dried ginger

1½ tsp. ground cumin

1½ tsp. ground coriander

½ tsp. paprika

¼ tsp. cayenne pepper

- Mix oil, orange juice, and spices together.
- Massage the mixture over the salmon, cover and refrigerate for 30 min.
- Grill or pan-sear for 3 min. skin side down, flip, and cook for an additional 3 min.
- Serve along with vegetables of choice.

DESSERT

While flax makes for a great, filling breakfast, chia has a unique consistency that lends itself to dessert puddings. Try these two and experiment with other ingredients.

PUMPKIN CHIA PUDDING

1½ cups soy or almond milk
½ cup pumpkin puree
1–2 scoops soy protein powder (optional)
1 tbsp. raw honey or agave nectar (optional)

1 tsp. vanilla extract
1 tsp. cinnamon
¼ tsp. nutmeg
⅛ tsp. ground ginger
⅛ tsp. ground cloves
¼ cup chia seeds

- Put all ingredients except chia into blender and blend until smooth.
- Transfer to a glass bowl and stir in chia seeds so they distribute evenly.
- Place in refrigerator for at least three hours.
- Serve and enjoy!

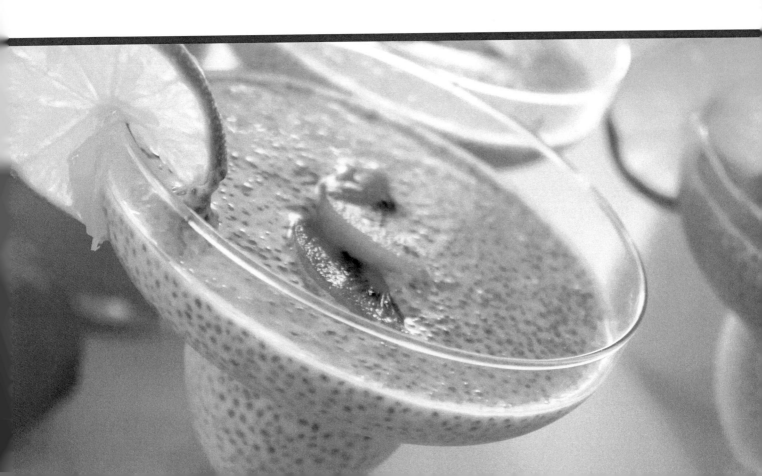

CHIA COCONUT PUDDING

12 oz. light coconut milk
⅓ cup chia seeds
¼ cup honey or agave nectar

1–2 scoops soy protein powder (optional)
Grated coconut, for garnish

- Blend all ingredients but chia and coconut shreds.
- Transfer to glass bowl and stir in chia seeds.
- Chill in the refrigerator for at least 3 hours. Serve garnished with shredded coconut.

John T., age 79

Dr. Dave's purpose is to extend our healthy lives. I was 78, quite overweight, had high blood pressure, drank a lot, slept poorly, and was badly out of shape physically. The first time I showed up at Dr. Dave's workout not only could I not do a sit-up but it took three people to boost me up off the mat!

When the group invited me to come back, I leaped at the opportunity to see what I could do. The hard work has paid off for me. I'm eating better, sleeping better, and moving better than I have in years. I have more strength, endurance, and flexibility. I've lost over 40 pounds.

Now I can get up off the mat without any assistance. I do sit-ups and push-ups with the rest of the guys, and even swing sledge hammers and flip large truck tires. My sense of well-being has improved. The enthusiasm is contagious; my wife Barbara, age 79, has even caught the habit. She too has lost weight and gained strength and endurance.

One of my greatest challenges is a fairly severe case of peripheral neuropathy, making it difficult to walk or to balance properly. I was amazed that Dr. Dave and his team wouldn't let me use this as an excuse to sit out even one exercise. They pushed me to do better and made an effort to modify each workout so that I could stay within my current capabilities. Even the best specialists have told me that there's nothing that modern medicine can offer to repair my nerve damage, but with this back-to-basics workout I'm moving better, balancing better, and I feel many times better than I did one year ago. I feel as though in the past 12 months I've gotten 10 years younger. I'm actually looking forward to seeing how I'm going to feel at eighty.

Dr. Dave exercises hard right along with his patients, encouraging us, down on the mat, lifting weights, flipping large truck tires, competing in team events and keeping a close eye on each of us. What a fine physician we are fortunate to have!

CHALLENGE #3: PLEASE DON'T PASS THE SALT

How sodium and potassium affect your health

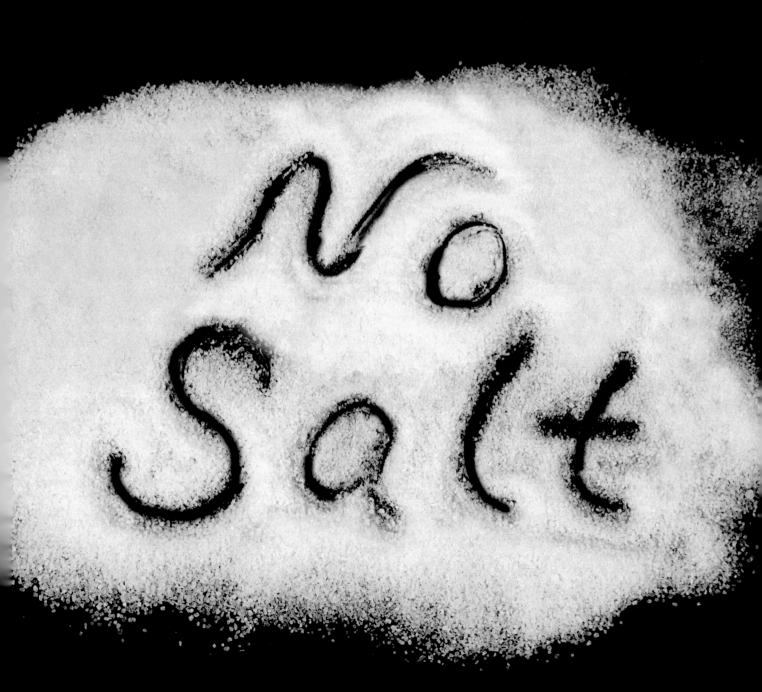

HIGH BLOOD PRESSURE IS ONE OF THE MOST COMMON MEDICAL CONDITIONS IN THE U.S., affecting a third of all adults, and nearly three-fourths of those over 75. There are a few lifestyle factors that impact blood pressure, but the most important by far is the balance of sodium and potassium in our diet. The effect of salt reduction can be extraordinarily powerful: I've seen my patients drop blood pressure medications only weeks after starting an exercise program and dropping salt from their diet. But sodium's effects don't stop at just blood pressure; excess sodium contributes to heart failure, kidney failure, kidney stones, and osteoporosis as well. If throwing away the salt shaker sounds hard, just think about how nice it would be to throw away your pills along with it.

SODIUM—WHAT IS IT GOOD FOR?

Sodium and potassium are two of the most important elements in the human body. Their balance across the membranes of our cells is what carries proteins, glucose, and other molecules in and out of our cells. Sodium also regulates nerve signals, including the sense of touch and pain. Billions of little chemical reactions each day rely on our having the right amount of sodium and potassium on board.

Your total body levels of sodium and potassium are roughly equivalent, but they aren't all in the same place. All the potassium in your body is sequestered inside your cells and all the sodium is outside the cells in your bloodstream. If you look at your last laboratory report from the doctor's office you'll see that the normal range for sodium is around 140 while the range for potassium is about 4. If we were able to test the fluid inside one of your cells we'd see the exact opposite, with a super-high potassium level and very little sodium. Little pumps along the cell membrane work nonstop to push sodium out of cells and keep potassium in. Other gates in the cell membrane will allow the sodium back in only if it comes along with certain other molecules, like glucose, for example. If a cell needs more glucose for energy it opens a channel that lets sodium rush in, carrying glucose along with it.

Maintaining the right levels of sodium and potassium is critical to our health. Not only do we need to get enough of each in our diet but we also need to get rid of any excess beyond what we need. This job is handled by our kidneys. If sodium levels in the body are low, the kidney tries to hold onto as much as possible, and if we have more than we need, the kidneys filter out the excess into the urine. The same goes for potassium—ingest too much and the excess ends up in the urine, ingest too little and the filter reverses to retain as much as possible.

But your kidney isn't just there to regulate sodium and potassium, of course; it has plenty of other functions as well. The kidney also regulates other important electrolytes like calcium, magnesium, and phosphate, all of which are important for bone health. It helps to regulate your acid balance by excreting the right amount of hydrogen and bicarbonate ions. Your kidneys also secrete hormones that control the amount of oxygen-carrying red blood cells in your body and other hormones, including renin and angiotensin that are critical for regulating blood pressure.

ON-THE-JOB TRAINING

Your kidneys clearly have a number of important jobs to do, and those jobs were defined by millions of years of evolution. Our kidneys developed their highly specialized filtration abilities in response to the demands of a hunter-gatherer diet. Any significant deviation from that ancestral diet has the potential to wreak havoc with our kidneys, especially if that deviation involves the two most important electrolytes in our bodies. Unfortunately, today's modern diet has the natural ratios of sodium and potassium turned upside down, making life for our kidneys very difficult indeed.

Back before the Agricultural Era, the only sodium in our diet was what was naturally available in the wild. Our ancestors had no way to add salt to the diet—when was the last time you stumbled upon salt on a nature hike? It wasn't until the Agricultural Era that we started using salt as a preservative and to enhance the flavor of food.

Prior to agriculture our ancestors had a much different problem from the one we have today—not enough salt. As crazy as that sounds, there's actually very little sodium in most natural foods. A serving of broccoli, for example, has only about 60 milligrams of sodium. A quarter pound of ground beef (grass-fed, of course) has about the same. Most other foods are in the same range, with a typical serving size accounting for about 50-60 milligrams of sodium at most. So eating 10-12 servings of anything would barely get you to 500 milligrams of sodium per day. This is probably about the amount that our ancestors had in their diets.

Looking way back to the very first days of mankind puts the salt equation in even more dramatic context. Humanity originated in Africa, which even back then was a hot and dry continent. Our ancestors thus had limited access to sodium and had the added challenge of trying not to sweat it all out by lunchtime. Think about how little sodium there is in natural foods, how arid the deserts can be, and how salty our sweat is. Our ancestors had to have an amazing ability to retain as much sodium as they could find in the diet. Consequently, we developed not only a refined taste for salt (it's no coincidence that this is by far the world's most popular spice and food additive) but also an evolutionary ability to retain sodium and water with great efficiency.

Natural foods may have very little sodium, but they do have a ton of potassium. A typical serving of any natural food has anywhere from 200-400 milligrams of potassium on average—about 5 to 10 times the amount of sodium. Potassium is found in more than just bananas; nearly every food group, including meats, nuts, fruits, and vegetables, has an abundance of potassium.

Quick tip: **Coconut water** *is low in calories and offers 400 milligrams or more of potassium per 8 ounce serving*

Ratio of potassium to sodium in natural foods

	Potassium	Sodium	Ratio
1 cup cooked beet greens	1,309	347	4:1
1 cup prunes	1,274	3	425:1
1 cup cooked soybeans	970	25	39:1
¼ cup tomato paste	670	39	17:1
¼ pound salmon	490	44	11:1
1 cup broccoli	457	64	7:1
1 sweet potato	438	72	6:1
1 medium banana	422	1	422:1
¼ pound lean ground beef	346	66	5:1
1 cup kale	296	30	10:1
1 tablespoon molasses	293	7	42:1
¼ pound chicken breast	256	74	3:1
½ cup walnuts	221	1	221:1
1 pear	206	2	103:1
1 apple	195	2	98:1
1 cup blueberries	114	1	114:1
1 egg	69	71	1:1
Total	8,026	849	9:1

Pay attention to the distinction between sodium and salt. Table salt is what we call sodium chloride, about 40% of which by weight is sodium. So 400 milligrams of sodium is equivalent to 1,000 milligrams of table salt.

THAT'S NOT IN MY JOB DESCRIPTION

Fast-forward to today and we see that our kidneys, highly specialized to retain sodium and excrete potassium, are faced with the exact opposite task on a daily basis. The typical American has close to 10,000 milligrams of salt each day, roughly 5x what our ancestors enjoyed, while also getting a lot less potassium. You might already guess that foods like pizza or fast food are loaded with salt, but it might surprise you to see just how much. For example, one personal pan pizza has more sodium than an entire week's food from a hunter-gatherer diet. Indulging just once or twice a month is enough to double or triple your sodium intake without your even knowing it.

Ratio of sodium to potassium in modern foods

	Sodium	Potassium	Ratio
12" hand-tossed pizza	5,055	1,277	4:1
Whopper with cheese	1,431	534	3:1
Medium French fries	326	546	1:1
Subway tuna sandwich (6 inch)	780	419	2:1
McDonald's Grilled Chicken Sandwich	820	456	2:1
Caesar salad with grilled chicken	580	755	1:1
Roasted Vegetable Pizza, Whole Wheat Crust	300	n/a	na
Amy's Light in Sodium Vegetable Lasagna	340	n/a	na
MorningStar soy breakfast patty	240	174	1:1
Gardenburger (chipotle flavor)	387	158	2:1
Triscuits (6)	216	108	2:1
Total	10,475	4,427	2:1

However, the big surprise is that many of the foods on the above table aren't junk food—they are low-calorie, organic, and even vegetarian options that most of us wouldn't think twice about buying. Two hundred milligrams of sodium per serving may not sound like much, but remember that that's not a whole meal, just a serving. For example, you're unlikely to make a meal out of a single Gardenburger without anything else on the side. Add up the servings and your healthy day can easily contain close to 10 grams of salt. Turn ahead to the end of the chapter to see a side-by-side comparison of a healthy American day and a healthy hunter-gatherer day. You'll see that you are clearly better off grabbing a handful of nuts or a piece of fruit than an organic, vegetarian, or whole wheat pizza any day of the week.

"Civilized" ratio of sodium to potassium

2:1

Hunter-gatherer ratio of sodium to potassium:

1:10

TURNING UP THE PRESSURE

Having your natural ratio of sodium and potassium turned upside down makes life pretty hard for your kidneys. Today they are asked to do a job for which they were never trained, plus multitask by managing your blood pressure as well. It's no surprise that the kidneys are not that great at pulling off this trick. Over time, blood pressure starts to creep up and eventually most of us end up with high blood pressure. Hypertension has now become the new normal.

Percentage of people in the U.S. with hypertension by age group

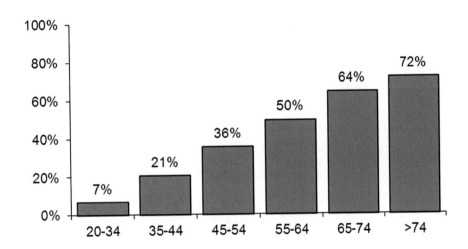

Studies on animals and humans consistently show that sodium excess and potassium deficiency are both highly correlated with high blood pressure. This research is hardly new; studies implicating sodium as a cause of hypertension date back over half a century. In fact, the INTERSALT study, which many experts would consider one of the landmark trials of sodium and hypertension, was published over twenty-five years ago.

The INTERSALT study compared blood pressure readings from over 10,000 members of different cultures from around the world and correlated them with dietary sodium and potassium intake. This trial is huge by any standard, with about ten times more people enrolled than in most large trials. People were enrolled from forty-eight urban centers around the world, as well as from four remote villages where people still lived off the land without access to modern foods (or salt).

Among the big cities, there was a clear correlation between sodium intake and high blood pressure. The study showed that an increase of about 2 grams of sodium per day would lead to an increase of about 6 points of blood pressure. Many other trials have found the same thing—what most people would consider to be a pretty significant reduction in salt intake leads to a relatively modest reduction in blood pressure. Dropping your blood pressure by 6 points probably won't get you off any of your medications for high blood pressure, making salt reduction a tough sell. This may be one reason that your doctor hasn't already pressed you to dramatically lower your sodium intake.

But there's more to this story. Getting rid of the excess sodium only solves half the problem for your kidneys; they also need more potassium. Solving the other half of the sodium/potassium imbalance doubles your reward; the amount of expected blood pressure reduction in this trial (and others) practically doubled when potassium intake increased along with the reduction in sodium. Increasing potassium by 4 grams per day in addition to reducing sodium by about 2 grams per day led to a 10 point reduction in blood pressure. Other studies have also shown that potassium from fruits and vegetables and even from supplements can lower blood pressure independent of the amount of sodium in the diet. These means that if you, like many other Americans, have 4 grams of excess sodium in your diet and are not getting enough potassium, you could expect to lower your blood pressure by between 10 to 15 points or more, simply by correcting the imbalance.

There are a few other factors that influence blood pressure, including drinking alcohol, being overweight, and not exercising enough. Improving all of these measures might get you another 5–10 points of blood pressure reduction above what you would get from optimizing your sodium and potassium. Depending on where you started you might be able

What causes high blood pressure?
- *Too much sodium*
- *Not enough potassium*
- *Too little exercise*
- *Weight gain*
- *Too much alcohol*

to lower your blood pressure by 30 points or more in a matter of weeks. Results like these are nothing short of amazing.

HYPERTENSION, THE PRICE OF BEING CIVILIZED

With up to 30 points or more of high blood pressure being attributable to lifestyle, it sounds like living like a hunter-gatherer may mean not having to deal with high blood pressure at all. If that's what you're thinking, you're right. There were four remote villages in the INTERSALT trial, including two in Brazil and one each in Kenya and New Guinea. These people lived thousands of miles from each other and shared no common ancestry; however, they did share some common characteristics—they lived off the land, had no or limited access to modern foods, and they consumed less than one gram of sodium a day on average. Basically, they followed the same diet we are learning about right here.

Of all the things these tribes had in common, the most impressive was that none of them got high blood pressure. Three of the villages—the two in Brazil and one in New Guinea—had no exposure at all to civilization. The Yanomamo tribe in Brazil did not have a single member with high blood pressure, while the Xingu tribe in Brazil and the tribe from New Guinea had a rate of hypertension of less than 1%. Compare that to America and other modern cultures where over 30% of adults have high blood pressure and you can see that there is something to living off the land.

In developed countries blood pressure rises with age, with people in their fifties having blood pressure about 15 points higher than those in their twenties. Not so in remote villages. Unlike in America or other civilized nations, these people did not see their blood pressure increase with age. Among the three villages with no exposure to civilization there was absolutely no increase in blood pressure with age. Nearly every villager studied had a blood pressure under 120/80, whether they were twenty or eighty years old.

Among the four villages, the one in Kenya was the only outlier with a 5% incidence of hypertension, still much less than the 30% in modern cultures. Not coincidentally, this village is the only one of the four that shared any traffic with a modernized city nearby, meaning that they had some regular exposure to a Western-type diet. Their blood pressure also had a slight increase with age that amounted to a couple of points per decade. They had a little salt in their diet and they had a little hypertension—just what you would expect.

Now just take a second to let this sink in: all evidence suggests that nearly every single case of high blood pressure can be attributed to our being outside of our natural habitat. We have become so used to our doctors putting us on blood pressure medications in our fifties and sixties that we just chalk it up to getting older. Who would believe that it's not getting older, but eating processed foods and sodium that gets you sicker? *You can get older without getting sicker.*

Americans with hypertension:	Hunter-gatherers with hypertension:
>30%	<5%

SO WHAT IF MY BLOOD PRESSURE GOES UP? IT HAPPENS TO EVERYBODY.

Having high blood pressure is a big deal. Just because everyone has it doesn't mean that it isn't important. Your blood pressure is akin to the oil pressure in your car—if you keep driving while the oil pressure light is on you'll wear out gaskets, break hoses, and eventually the whole car will break down. Ignore the light when the pressure gets *really* high and you might blow the engine before you even get back to the garage.

The same thing happens in your body. Your body is designed to work at a pressure below 120/80. Above this level the extra pressure wears out the blood vessels leading to the heart, kidney, brain, and other important organs. If the blood pressure is just a little too high, the damage takes longer to develop, and if the blood pressure reaches a critical level, you might actually burst a blood vessel. If that artery is in your brain, the damage can be severe or even fatal. Even without such dramatic events, high blood pressure is associated with strokes, heart attacks, and kidney failure. The scary thing is that all this happens without you feeling a thing until it's too late and the damage is done. This is why in medical circles we call hypertension the "silent killer."

Having untreated high blood pressure increases your risk of dying from a heart attack or stroke by anywhere from 200% to 10,000% (no, that's not a typo). Even on medication, most people with high blood pressure don't make it to an optimal 120/80. And even if the drugs do work, you can't completely medicate away the extra risk of organ damage or death. Even people with treated hypertension still have a higher risk of death than those with normal blood pressure off medications. To use the car analogy again, it's like continuing to drive your car with the oil pressure indicator flashing. You can change hoses and gaskets to keep up with the wear and tear but if you never fix the underlying problem, your car won't last as long as your neighbor's.

Most Americans will eventually die from cardiovascular disease, which is definitely not something to look forward to. Reducing your blood pressure by 20 points reduces your risk of death from any cause by over 25% over the following sixteen years, and lowers your risk of dying from cardiovascular disease by over one-third. Managing your blood pressure with diet and exercise could be the most important thing you ever do.

NO BONES ABOUT IT

Now let's move on past hypertension and talk about another important topic: your skeleton. If there is one condition that we universally equate with old age it has to be osteoporosis. While some young people struggle with diabetes, high cholesterol, and heart disease, there are few people with osteoporosis that don't also qualify for Medicare. At thirty-five or forty years old, our bones are tough and sturdy, but only a few decades later we risk a broken hip every time we step out of the shower or off a curb. Getting old is no picnic. But could it be possible that diet and exercise, rather than age alone, are to blame? You bet it is.

We all know that calcium and vitamin D are important for bone health. Your doctor probably tells you every year to make sure you get enough of both. But if everyone knows this, why do so many people have osteoporosis? It's probably because of all that sodium lurking in our healthy American diets.

It turns out that a low potassium, high sodium diet is not very healthy for your bones any more than it is for your blood pressure. Table salt is metabolized into acid, and it is probably the greatest contributor of acid in our diet. Your body doesn't do very well in an acidic environment—you may remember dissolving metal keys in your high school chemistry class in a plastic beaker full of acid. It should be common sense that anything that can eat through solid steel can't be good for our bodies. Our bodies will do just about anything to keep from getting too acidic, even if it means sacrificing one organ to save the whole.

In the case of an acidic diet, the casualty is your skeleton. Bone is a rich store of both calcium and phosphate. Phosphate is necessary for calcium to stay attached to bone; without phosphate there's no skeleton. Now, it just so happens that phosphate is also an excellent buffer that can be used to balance out the acid in your body. If your diet is too acidic, your body just pulls some phosphate away from the bone to buffer the acid in your blood. The more acidic the diet, the more phosphate comes leaching out of bone. Given enough time, your bones will slowly deteriorate no matter how much calcium and vitamin D you take every day, simply because there's not enough phosphate to glue calcium to bone, where it belongs.

THE NEW "STONE" AGE

But wait, it gets worse. Now that there's not enough phosphate in the bone, all that calcium has to go somewhere. If it can't form bone it just floats around until it reaches the kidneys, which are the filter for all the minerals in our blood. When the kidneys see your calcium levels rising they will just filter it out, which means more calcium in your bladder where it doesn't belong. Before you know it you've got calcium crystallizing into stones that bounce around until they get stuck and you end up in the emergency room with excruciating back pain. Ever have to pass a kidney stone? Gosh, I hope not.

THE END OF THE ROAD

Your poor kidneys try desperately your entire life to deal with this new high-sodium, low-potassium world they are in. Every day they do the job they were never designed to do, and over the years they get less and less successful at it. Your blood pressure rises, your bones melt away, and finally the kidney just starts to shut down. Over time and with age your kidneys start to fail, and even if you don't end up with osteoporosis or high blood pressure, you live long enough to see your kidneys go first. Over 15% of adults have some degree of kidney failure, with about 3% eventually requiring dialysis. High blood pressure and diabetes are the two most common causes of kidney failure, and reducing your sodium intake goes a long way to reducing your risk of needing dialysis someday.

Excess sodium is an acid
An acidic diet is linked to osteoporosis,
kidney stones, and kidney failure

HOW DO I KNOW IF I'VE GOT TOO MUCH ACID IN THE BLOOD?

Chances are you can't know. Your life depends on your blood not getting too acidic, so your kidneys will do anything to keep your acid balance in a very tight range. If you check your blood you'll find that your acid balance is near perfect, but that doesn't tell you anything. What matters is how your blood is getting that way. Is it because your diet is balanced or because every day a little more phosphate gets sucked out of your bones? Only you know the answer to that one; everyone else will have to wait to see whether your body starts to break down after another few decades.

However, there is one measure on routine blood work that correlates somewhat with the amount of acid in the diet: your chloride level. Chloride is commonly checked along with other liver and kidney tests as part of your annual physical. An elevated chloride level may indicate that your blood is starting to get too acidic and your kidneys are working overtime to maintain a neutral balance.

WHERE ELSE IS ACID CREEPING IN?

Salt isn't the only contributor of acid in our diet. Animal protein in meats, fish, and dairy all gets metabolized into acid in our body. Cheese is acidic, because it contains both animal protein and salt. Many diet drinks and sodas are also highly acidic. Diet and regular sodas, which contain both sodium and phosphoric acid, have an acidity level approaching that of stomach acid.

Acidity levels of common beverages compared to stomach acid

	pH
Stomach acid	1.5
Arizona Iced Tea	2.9
Diet Pepsi	2.9
Diet Dr. Pepper	3.0
Diet Coca-Cola	3.2
Diet Mountain Dew	3.3
Diet Sprite	3.3
Brewed Black Tea	5.4
Brewed Black Coffee	6.3
Water	6.7

On the pH scale an increase in 1 unit corresponds to a 10-fold increase in acidity. For example, stomach acid is about 10x more acidic than Arizona Iced Tea, which is about 1,000x more acidic than brewed coffee.

BACK TO BASIC

Clearly, we want to start to get away from having such an acidic diet. The first part of the solution is getting rid of all that excess sodium. Avoid most sauces, condiments, and gravies. Eliminating the most acidic beverages, primarily bottled sodas, is the next step. Now all we need to do is find something to eat that can cancel out all the acid in meat protein.

Luckily for us, meat protein is the only part of the caveman diet that gets metabolized into acid in our bodies. The protein in animal products has a sulfur molecule attached, which is metabolized into sulfuric acid when digested. Vegetable proteins have no sulfur and so do not increase the amount of acid in the body. Nuts, legumes, vegetables, and fruits are all basic (the opposite of acidic). You can get up to one-third or one-half the calories in your diet from meat and still stay neutral to basic if you get the rest of your calories from all-natural foods. There's no need to become a vegetarian, but you do need to get enough plants to balance out your acid load from meat.

Acidic	Basic
Meat	Fruits
Dairy	Vegetables
Salt	Nuts
Soda	Legumes

Eliminate the added sodium, lose the diet soda, and eat more veggies. That's all there is to it. You'll drastically reduce the amount of work your kidneys are required to do to keep your blood chemistry properly balanced. Phosphate can go back into the bone where it belongs and you'll pass every bone density test with flying colors. Your blood pressure may drop substantially, and your kidneys will be sure to last a lifetime. Easy enough.

BUT I CAN'T HELP MYSELF

Well, maybe not quite. You might say that you love salt and you don't want to give it up. News flash—neither does anyone else. Your passion for salt is a survival technique from days long past. Remember how scarce sodium is in the real world? It's only natural that we would evolve to crave sodium and consume it every chance we get. You're hardwired down to your bones to start salivating anytime somebody waves a salt-crusted pretzel or a sodium-laden burger your way. There's a reason McDonald's and Burger King make so much money.

This isn't conjecture; it's a well-studied fact. Modern studies consistently support the fact that humans are helpless when it comes to craving salt. The only time we don't eat it is when we can't get it. When salt is introduced into an unsuspecting population the taste for it readily increases (think about those Kenyan villagers who saw their blood pressures start to rise with even a little exposure to sodium in the diet). About 20% of people will salt food even before they taste it. When research-ers sneakily change the size of the pores in salt shakers, most people don't notice the difference; the amount of shaking is independent of the amount of salt that comes out. Salt comes out and we grab it without a second thought.

But this story isn't all doom and gloom. Just because you are hardwired to eat salt doesn't mean you have to. Lab rats don't have the good sense to delay gratification, but we do. You would probably have rather slept in, surfed, and played outside for the past twenty years but instead you sucked it up and worked all day. You've proven your ability to put aside your pleasure today in order to earn a better tomorrow. You can do the same thing here. Put aside your guilty pleasure and the immediate gratifi-cation of a salted palate in favor of a less medicated, healthier body tomorrow.

As hard as it might be to start cutting back, it will get easier with time. Studies show that even salt junkies begin to lose their taste for salt after just a few weeks. After a couple of months on a low-sodium diet, most people rate salty and un-salty foods the same on an enjoyment scale. The food and drug industries may have you hooked, but it only takes a few weeks to be free of their clutches, so hang in there and you'll be okay.

HUNTING FOR SALT AND GATHERING POTASSIUM

Let's start by looking at where the sodium lurks in your diet. The chances are that less than 20% of the sodium in your diet comes from your own cooking or the salt you add at the table. Most studies suggest that 10% comes from your compulsive salt shaking and another 10% from that pinch of salt or baking soda you add to everything in the kitchen. I would definitely recommend starting here with your salt reduction efforts. Twenty percent might not sound like much, but it is the part that is easiest to cut back on and will get you one-fifth of the way there. If you are getting 10 grams of salt in your daily diet, then there's 2 grams right here that are easy pickings.

The other 80% or more comes from the food made by others; eating out at restaurants or eating packaged foods. Read any label and you will see that there is no way to avoid sodium when eating anything out of a box. The fact that people love salt has not been lost on anyone in the food business. If I open a restaurant, my main goal is to sell food, not save lives. Consequently, it behooves me to put as much salt in the food as possible. A research study published in *The Journal of the American Medical Association* found that sodium levels in restaurant foods average about 500 milligrams of sodium (equivalent to about ½ teaspoon of salt) in a quarter pound serving of food. If you figure the average portion of food at a sitting is closer to half a pound (sandwich and side, for example), then the amount of sodium you get per meal is probably closer to 1,000 milligrams or a full teaspoon of salt. Eat out more than once a week without paying attention to this and your efforts at preventing sodium-related diseases are likely to be in vain.

Success depends on your thinking like a hunter-gatherer. Definitely stop eating packaged foods. If you are in an absolute bind then avoid anything with over 100 milligrams of sodium and anything that has more sodium than potassium. Trust me; this doesn't leave many packaged-food options. Assume that any pre-made food that isn't labeled salt-free has the average 500 milligrams sodium per ¼ pound serving. This goes for anything at the deli counter or pre-made dinners at the local grocer (yes, even the organic ones).

When eating out you'll want to be a stickler for sodium. Assume that restaurants will put as much salt into food as they can get away with. Sometimes it's tough to take a stand on sodium; nobody wants to be "that guy" who can't go anywhere out to eat without making a huge production out of ordering a meal. Well, "that guy" is the guy who also doesn't take any medications and will probably outlive everyone else at the table. My wife is already used to the fact that it takes me longer to order at most restaurants than it does most people to open a brokerage account. She deals with my zealous avoidance of salt, and your family will too. Avoid sauces and condiments, all of which are just different guises for the same sodium that's in the salt shaker.

If dropping sodium still sounds dire, ease the blow by reserving a day or two a month to enjoy a good meal out on the town. Your body can handle the occasional dose of sodium, just not the daily barrage that it has probably been getting for the past several decades.

Challenge #3: Put down the salt shaker and start counting the sodium and potassium in your diet. For the next two weeks limit your daily sodium to less than 1,000 milligrams and try to get at least 4,000 milligrams of potassium daily from all-natural sources.

I've found through experience that blood pressure tends to be one of the first things to respond dramatically to my diet and exercise program. Many of my patients lower their blood pressure medications within the first several weeks. So set the bar high and really nail this challenge right!

"Healthy" American day	Sodium (mg)	Potassium (mg)
Breakfast, Turkey bacon breakfast sandwich		
Turkey bacon, 1 oz.	366	63
Whole wheat English muffin	240	139
1 large egg	71	69
1 slice low fat cheese	56	31
Lunch, Turkey sandwich with low-fat cheese on whole wheat bread		
Wheat bread, 2 slices	291	163
Turkey, 6 slices	854	170
Low-fat Swiss cheese, 2 slices	111	62
1 tbsp. mustard	170	21
Midday snack		
Pure Protein power bar	190	145
Dinner, Whole wheat pasta with organic marinara sauce and lean ground-turkey		
1 cup whole wheat pasta	62	4
1 cup organic tomato sauce	940	900
¼ lb. ground turkey	51	295
Side salad with low-fat dressing		
1 cup lettuce	10	70
Reduced fat thousand island dressing, 1 tbsp.	143	30
Dessert		
4 Famous Amos chocolate chip cookies	104	53
Total milligrams	3,659	2,062
Milligrams of salt	9,148	
Ratio of sodium to potassium	**1.8:1**	

Healthy hunter-gatherer day	Sodium (mg)	Potassium (mg)
Spinach omelet with side of berries		
2 large omega-3 eggs	142	138
1 egg white	55	54
1 cup spinach, sautéed in olive oil	126	839
1 cup of blueberries	1	114
Midmorning snack		
40 almonds	0	352
Lunch, Grilled chicken with leftover curried okra		
Curried okra, 2 cups	19	432
¼ lb. grilled chicken breast	77	247
Midday snack		
Kale chips, 2 cups (no salt added)	51	658
Apple, large, with skin	2	239
Dinner		
Salmon fillet, 4 oz.	134	408
Grilled asparagus, 12 spears	5	484
Mashed sweet potatoes, 1 cup	72	950
Dessert		
Dark chocolate, 1 oz.	7	158
Asian pear	0	333
Total milligrams	691	5,406
Milligrams of salt	1,728	
Ratio of sodium to potassium	**1:7.8**	

BREAKFAST

KALE & COCONUT SMOOTHIE

½ cup coconut milk
2 cups of chopped kale or spinach
1 ripe banana or half an avocado
½ cup pineapple, drained

- Add coconut milk to blender followed by other ingredients. Blend until smooth, adding water as needed.

VERY BERRY KALE & FLAX SMOOTHIE

2 cups chopped kale
2 tbsp. ground flax seed
½ cup coconut milk or soy milk
1 banana, raw or frozen, chopped
1 cup frozen berries

- Add coconut milk to blender followed by other ingredients. Blend until smooth, adding water as needed.

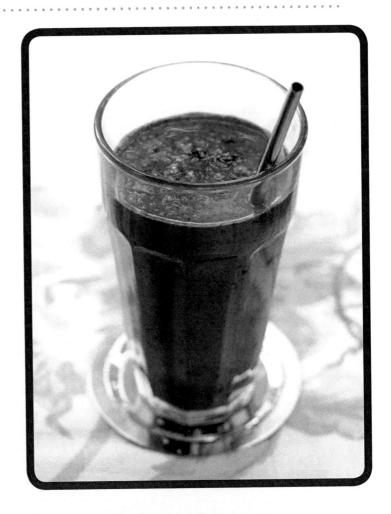

CHOCOLATE BANANA MUFFINS

3 very ripe bananas
2 tbsp. coconut oil, melted
¼ cup honey or maple syrup
1 large omega-3 egg
1 tsp. vanilla extract

1 cup almond meal
¼ cup coconut flour
⅓ cup unsweetened cocoa
¼ cup chopped nuts

- Preheat oven to 350°F. Line a muffin tin with liners.
- Mash bananas in large bowl, then mix in wet ingredients until thoroughly combined.
- Add flour and other dry ingredients and mix thoroughly.
- Scoop batter into muffin liners and sprinkle additional nuts on top.
- Bake 18 minutes, or until a toothpick comes out clean.

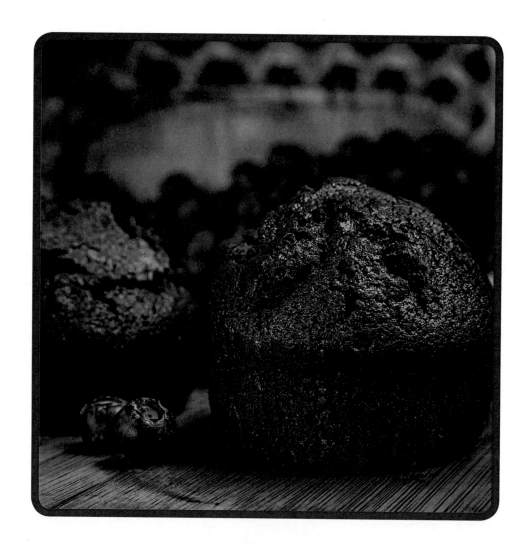

CONDIMENTS

Just because you're throwing away the salt doesn't mean your taste buds have to suffer. Try a few of these recipes for homemade condiments that won't raise your blood pressure.

MUSTARD

½ cup mustard powder
½ cup water

- Mix thoroughly in a bowl.
- Allow to settle for 15–20 minutes.
- Store refrigerated in sealed container.

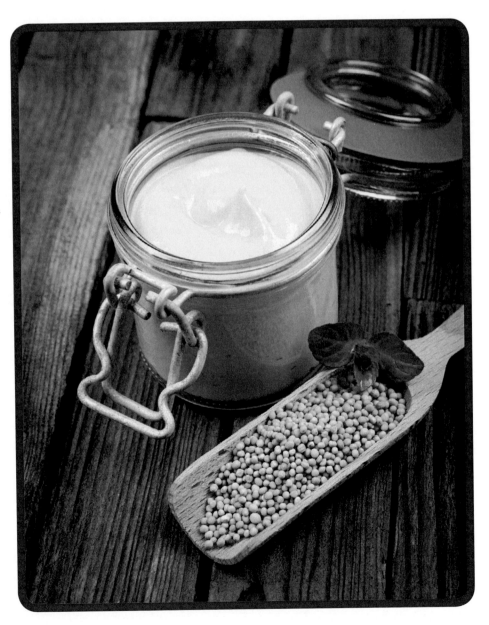

KETCHUP (ADAPTED FROM ULTIMATEPALEOGUIDE.COM)

2 6 oz. cans tomato paste
1 cup of vegetable broth
¼ cup apple cider vinegar

1 tbsp. of onion powder
1 tbsp. of garlic powder
¾ tsp. allspice

- Combine all ingredients thoroughly in small saucepan.
- Simmer over medium-low heat for 10 minutes.
- Allow to cool and store refrigerated in sealed container.

KETCHUP (ADAPTED FROM PALEOTABLE.COM)

1 15 oz. can tomato sauce (salt-free)
6 oz. can tomato paste
1 tbsp. apple cider vinegar
¾ tsp. garlic powder

¼ tsp. onion powder
¼ tsp. allspice
⅛ tsp. ground cloves

- Combine all ingredients thoroughly in small saucepan.
- Simmer over medium-low heat for 10 minutes.
- Allow to cool and store refrigerated in sealed container.

HOMEMADE BBQ SAUCE (ADAPTED FROM VAHUNTERGATHERERS.COM)

½ cup homemade ketchup
2 tbsp. blackstrap molasses
1 tbsp. apple cider vinegar
1 tbsp. mustard powder

¾ tsp. chili powder
½ tsp. ancho chili powder
½ tsp. paprika
¼ tsp. black pepper

- Combine all ingredients in mixing bowl, mix thoroughly with whisk.
- Allow to sit for at least 30 minutes. Store refrigerated in sealed container.

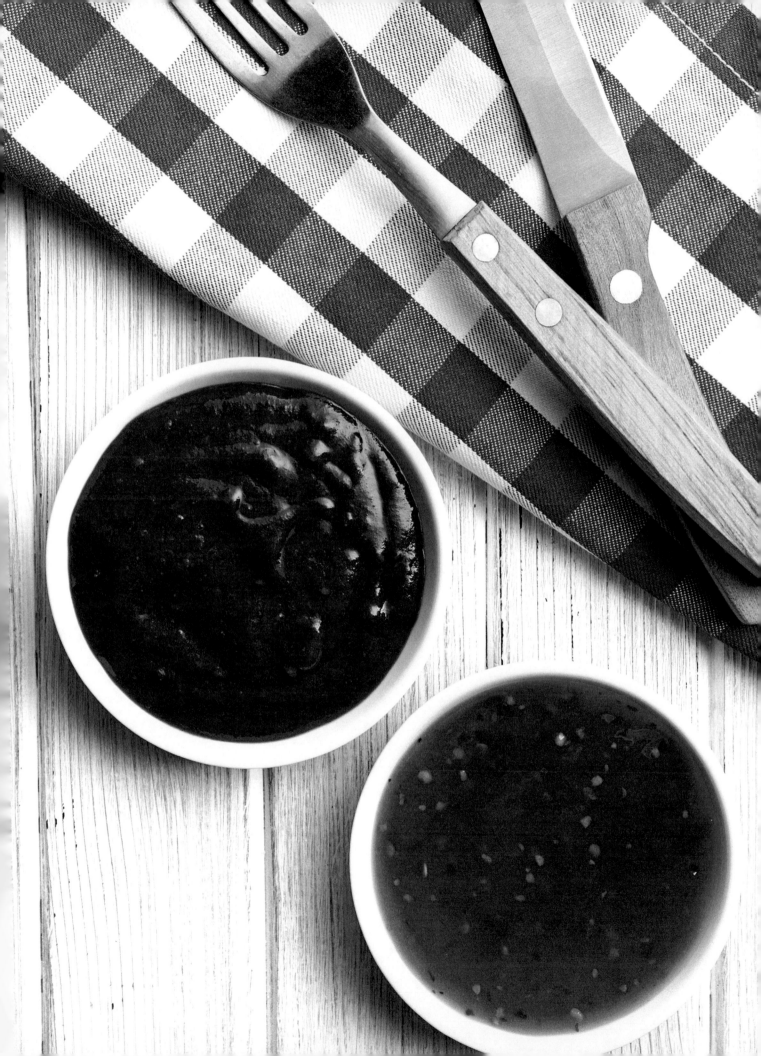

LUNCH, DINNER & SIDES

ROASTED BEETS WITH SAUTÉED BEET GREENS (ADAPTED FROM ALLRECIPES.COM)

1 bunch beets with greens
¼ cup olive oil
2 cloves garlic, minced

2 tbsp. chopped onion
1 tbsp. red wine vinegar

- Preheat oven to 350°F.
- Wash beets and greens thoroughly, remove greens and set aside.
- Toss beets with 2 tbsp. olive oil in large baking dish.
- Cover and bake for 45 to 60 minutes or until tender.
- While beets are cooking, heat remaining olive oil in skillet over medium heat.
- Sauté garlic and onion for 2 minutes or until fragrant.
- Chop or tear greens into 2–3 inch pieces and add to hot skillet.
- Remove from heat after greens are wilted.
- Serve beets drizzled with vinegar or alone. Serve greens alongside beets.

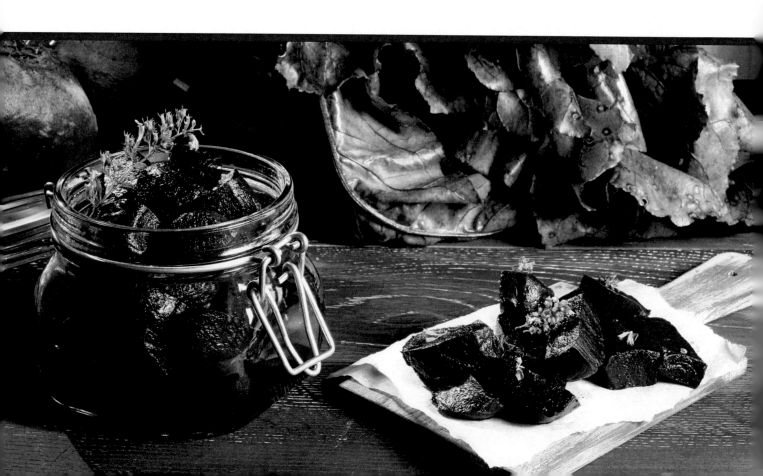

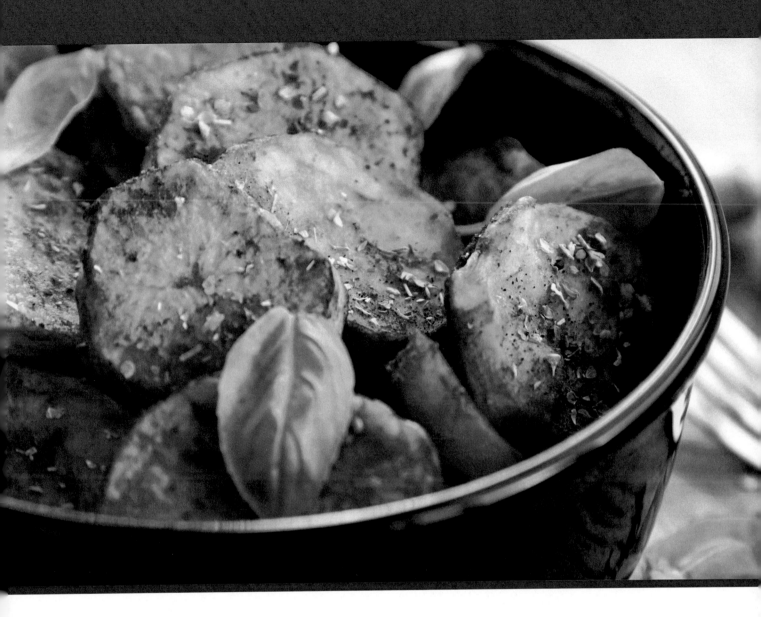

SWEET POTATO CHIPS

1 large sweet potato
Olive oil

Salt-free seasoning

- Preheat oven to 400°F.
- Slice sweet potato into rounds about ¼ inch thick.
- Brush with olive oil and arrange on baking sheet.
- Cook for 15 minutes, turning halfway through.

DESERTS

PRUNES STEWED IN PORT WINE (ADAPTED FROM THEKITCHN.COM)

½ pound dried prunes
1 clementine, sliced very thin
1 cinnamon stick

½ tsp. ground nutmeg
1 cup ruby port
2 tbsp. blackstrap molasses

- Combine all the ingredients in a 2-quart saucepan.
- Add enough water to bring the liquid level just up over the prunes.
- Bring to a simmer and cook, uncovered, over medium-low heat for about half an hour, or until the prunes are very soft.
- Add more water as it simmers, if necessary.

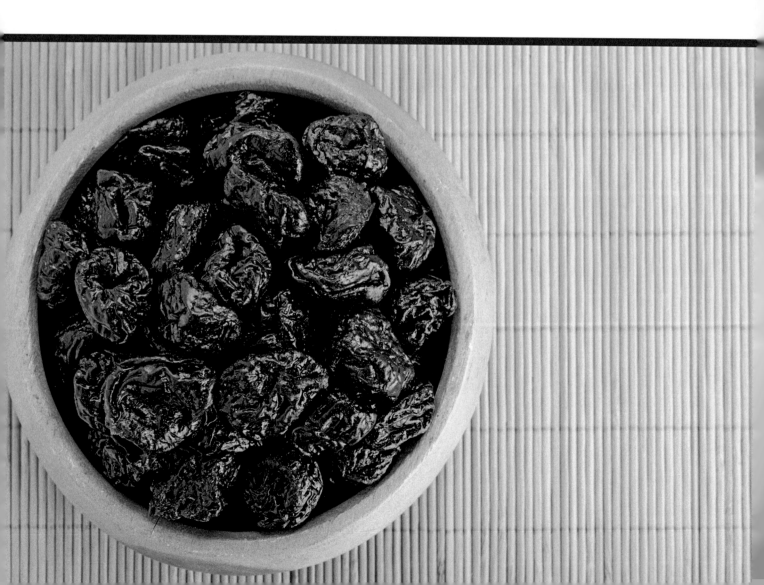

Mark S., age 69

I began seeing Dr. Dave in early 2012. As did my previous doctor, he asked for a fasting blood test, which I did. I had been on an ever-increasing spiral of high blood pressure and high blood sugars, with more medications getting added every year. When my hemoglobin A1c reached 8.2 Dr. Dave informed me that the only medication left to add was insulin. My dad took insulin and I was not particularly interested in doing so myself.

This was when he told me about his experiment of putting diet and exercise to the test. The other volunteers were just like me; men about my age who were having some of the same problems that I was. I jumped at the chance.

The thought of going on a hunter-gatherer diet along with a good workout didn't sound tough for an 18-year-old but I was well out of that age group. I did like the idea of working out since I had spent over 20 years in the military, but I hadn't done any exercising for over 15 years.

Changing my diet has been hard but over time it's gotten easier. I can't tell the taste of grass-fed beef from any other kind but I am eating a lot more vegetables and I am working on finding better meat. I eat more fish and I haven't had ice cream for a long time. My weight is down from 220 to a respectable 182 pounds. I am not having any problems with cheating, just with making sure I am eating a good, balanced meal.

I have been taken off one of my blood pressure pills and my blood pressure seems to sit at around 125/70. I hope that I will be reducing my pill intake again soon. My hemoglobin A1c has come down from 8.2 to 6.3 without any medication at all.

My blood sugars are down significantly and my kidney function is actually improving. As you can see, I have a way to go but my numbers are improving. I have spent 68 years building up these numbers and seeing these results after a year's work is pretty amazing. I have made no changes other than working at better eating and exercise. I can't tell you how happy I am and look forward to continued improvements with the next set of tests.

I have also noted another improvement—one I hadn't even considered until after I started the exercise program. On my first day of working out, I couldn't even do the warm-up exercises without holding on to a rope or wall for stability. Now they are natural to me without any added support. Remembering that as people get older the impact of falls is significant, I think that Dr. Dave has taken me from a potential serious fall risk to not being concerned with it at all.

I wholeheartedly support what Dr. Dave presents in his book and intend to continue to be an active participant in his program.

CHALLENGE #4: FIBER—IT'S NOT JUST ABOUT BEING REGULAR

YES, YOU ALREADY KNOW THAT FIBER IS GOOD FOR YOU. No news there. You may even think that you already get plenty of fiber. But even after getting this far in the Challenges, my guess is that you're still not getting nearly enough fiber to really move the needle on your health. Surprised? Don't be. Even the healthiest eaters rarely get to a healthy level of fiber intake without making a conscious and educated effort, and that's exactly what this Challenge is all about. By the time we're done I promise that you'll understand not only how much fiber you should be getting but also why you need it and how you can get it.

THE FIBER PRIMER

Let's begin with a quick primer on fiber and how it is different from everything else we eat. Fiber is a type of complex carbohydrate, not unlike what you would find in a piece of bread or a bowl of pasta. Most carbohydrate is in the form of long chains of simple sugars like fructose and glucose that are linked by chemical bonds. These large molecules are too big to pass through the intestinal wall and have to be broken down by enzymes secreted by our salivary glands and pancreas before they can be absorbed. Our enzymes are very efficient at breaking up most carbohydrates in our diet, but not fiber.

Fiber is also made up of individual sugar molecules; the difference is in the bonds between them. Fiber molecules contain bonds that cannot be broken by the enzymes in our digestive tract. Unable to be broken down into the small bits of glucose and fructose that we can absorb, these long chains of sugar pass right by the small intestine and aren't absorbed along with the rest of the food.

There are two types of fiber: soluble and insoluble. Both are found throughout the plant world in seeds, nuts, grains, fruits, and vegetables. Insoluble fiber is like tree bark; it can be ground up but won't dissolve in water. Instead it just gets carried right through your intestines like a leaf in a stream.

Soluble fiber, on the other hand, dissolves in our digestive tract, turning what was once watery liquid into a thick, viscous solution much like Jell-O. It is this thickening action that accounts for most of the health benefits of fiber. The Jell-O-like matrix created by the dissolved fiber traps water and small particles, affecting the way food is absorbed and the way our stools pass through the colon. This simple chemistry trick has an outsized effect when it comes to living a long time free of disease.

If you want to see this for yourself, just mix two tablespoons of psyllium husks in about six ounces of water and let it sit for a few hours. It won't be long before a spoon will stand straight up in the middle of the glass.

BIG PHARMA WISHES THEY HAD THOUGHT OF THIS...

Trapping water and small particles doesn't sound like much, but it turns out that turning water into Jell-O is like getting three or four medications rolled into one. For starters, both soluble and insoluble fiber help bind up sugar and other carbohydrates so they take longer to make it to the intestinal wall to get absorbed. The more fiber you eat, the less rapidly sugars are absorbed, leading to less insulin production. Less insulin production is good—our bodies were never meant to have chronically high levels of insulin production. People who have more fiber consequently have a lower risk of developing diabetes. This matters even if you don't have diabetes right now. The incidence of diabetes increases from only 4% for people under 45 to over 25% for those over 65, making this one of the most important age-related medical problems that isn't really age-related.

Fiber also does a good job of trapping cholesterol in its gelatinous matrix, thereby preventing its absorption. Cholesterol is important—we need it to live. Cholesterol makes our cell membranes nice and fluid and is the backbone of important hormones like estrogen and testosterone. However, as we learned in Challenge #2, most of the cholesterol made by our livers is sent to one place—our gallbladder. Cholesterol in the gallbladder is stored in the form of bile salts, which are released into the intestines every time we have a fatty meal. The bile salts help break up fats into individual triglycerides for absorption, similar to the way other enzymes break up carbohydrates into simple sugars. Once their job is done the bile salts are reabsorbed along with their cholesterol further down in the intestines.

Cholesterol has a number of important jobs, but as we know, too much of a good thing can lead to trouble. High cholesterol levels, of LDL in particular, are linked to heart attacks and strokes. Here's where fiber comes in. Fiber interferes with the usual gallbladder–cholesterol cycle by binding up the bile salts (and any cholesterol in your meal). Instead of getting reabsorbed, the bile and cholesterol just go right through you. This means that less cholesterol is around to clog up your arteries.

With enough fiber in the diet, cholesterol levels can drop significantly. In fact, studies suggest that increasing your fiber intake to levels our ancestors enjoyed can lower cholesterol by up to 25%. This is on a par with what you would get from a starting dose of Lipitor or other cholesterol medications, making you wonder how many people could get off medications for cholesterol simply by eating like a hunter-gatherer.

Interestingly, the heart-protecting benefits of fiber seem to go well beyond its cholesterol-lowering effect. Even modest increases in fiber intake, in the order of only a few grams daily, can reduce your risk of dying from heart disease by up to 25%. More fiber gets you even better results—a study published in the top medical journal, *The Lancet*, showed that men who got the least dietary fiber were 4x more likely to die from heart disease than those who got the most fiber. That's roughly equivalent to a 75% reduction in risk of death. If fiber were a drug, these are the kinds of numbers that would have pharmaceutical execs running to pick out a new private jet.

A high-fiber diet is associated with a 25% reduction in cholesterol and up to a 75% reduction in risk of death from heart disease.

PARDON ME, THAT'S JUST MY COLONOSCOPE YOU'RE FEELING

Fiber has far-reaching effects throughout the body, but some of fiber's greatest health benefits occur right there in your colon. Colon health is super-important; in fact, getting your colonoscopy is a rite of passage marking the official and inglorious start of being middle-aged. It's one of the first indignities we're forced to suffer with aging and lands right on that 50th birthday when you can no longer kid yourself that you're a young guy or girl anymore.

Ever since Katie Couric put her colon out for public display on *The Today Show*, the colonoscopy experience has become an acceptable subject of conversation over dinner or on the golf course. But for all the talk about colonoscopies, have you ever given much thought to why we are doing them?

We do this test for the simple reason that colon cancer is one of the most common cancers in America, and it is treatable if caught early with that colonoscopy. We do the colonoscopy, look for precancerous polyps, and snip them out before they turn really bad. If we find a polyp, you're likely to be asked to come back for another colonoscopy in as little as three years instead of the usual ten. But for all the money, time, and suffering we spend on colon cancer screening, no one ever asks why colon cancer is so common in the first place.

I'll give you a hint: getting a high-fiber diet can lower your risk of getting colon cancer by about 70%. If fiber were a drug this would be yet another statistic that would have pharma execs wringing their hands in glee. Colon cancer, believe it or not, is another disease that is associated with a Western-style low-fiber diet. The rates of colon polyps and colon cancer in the U.S. are about 10x those of developing countries in Asia and Africa. If you think that might be genetics, think again. The Japanese have one of the lowest rates of colon cancer in the world, but one generation after moving to America their rates of colon cancer are the same as ours. It's not the genetics; it's that low-fiber diet.

So now we've got two lethal diseases—colon cancer and heart disease—that are two of the most common causes of death for men and women over fifty in this country and both are inextricably linked to our low-fiber diet. By now you might be glazing over at all these numbers, but take a minute to step back and think about what this means to you. Through one simple step—increasing your fiber intake—you can cut your risk of dying from two of the most common killers in old age by 70%. Picture standing in a room at age seventy with nine other people; then at age eighty only three of you are left. Wouldn't you want to be one of those three? *Fiber helps you live longer.*

A high fiber diet reduces your risk of colon cancer by 70%

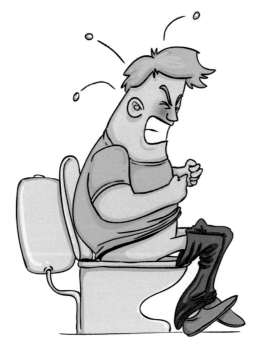

LIVE LONG AND PROSPER

Not only are you likely to live longer, but you will probably live better. Let's start with one thing that you probably took for granted in your younger years—the joy of taking a proper poop. Studies suggest that up to one-third of adults, or over 63 million Americans, suffer from constipation, and that number goes up with age. Fiber is the easy solution, but you don't want to wait until you're on the john pushing so hard your eyes feel like they're going to pop out of your head to start adding it to the routine. Many people wait until that very moment before the thought of fiber crosses their minds, but by then it's too late. Think of fiber as maintenance for your plumbing, not a quick fix. All that fiber in your system retains water, and with plenty of water and fiber running through your system, your plumbing will keep on working just fine. A high-fiber diet moves through your system about 30% faster than a low-fiber diet. Over time that means the difference between being stopped up and being on the go.

All that straining has another unpleasant effect often chalked up to age—hemorrhoids. The same mechanics of a low-fiber diet that contribute to constipation also lead to hemorrhoids. When you are straining, or the stool is hard and backed up in your colon, blood that circulates to the colon wall can flow down to the rectum but then can't easily flow back around. Just like varicose veins in your legs, the blood vessels in the rectum swell up and can become clotted and inflamed, eventually turning into hemorrhoids. Hemorrhoids are painful, uncomfortable, and embarrassing. No one wants to deal with them at home, much less have to end up bending over in the doctor's office with their pants around their ankles looking for a solution. Better to just get your fiber and keep your pants on.

But wait, there's more. There's yet another colon problem that we run into as we age—diverticulitis. If you've heard of it, you know how bad it can get. If you haven't, then pay attention. You'll thank me.

Your colon is made up of two walls; the inner wall that absorbs water and a muscular outer wall that squeezes everything in the right direction. When you leave your natural habitat and start consuming a low-fiber diet, you don't have enough water in the colon to keep everything moving. This creates uneven spots where the muscles get stuck—think of trying to squeeze out a tube of toothpaste with a lump of dried toothpaste inside. You would have to put more pressure on some areas and less on others, rather than just gradually squeezing from the bottom up.

When your colon has to squeeze harder and unevenly, bad things start to happen. Those muscles start to separate, and the soft inner wall then actually gets squeezed out into your abdomen, creating pockets that stick out from the colon wall. It is as though you were squeezing a balloon in your fist and watching the thin skin of the balloon pop out between your fingers. Your colon's inner wall isn't made to float around in your abdomen outside the protection of the muscular layer. These pockets fill up with stool, get inflamed and start causing chronic pain. Eventually they can rupture, which can be catastrophic.

This may sound esoteric but diverticulosis is actually one of the most common age-related diseases. If you are over fifty and you don't have it, you probably know someone who does. One-third of people over fifty have diverticulosis. In our seventies the rate goes up to 50%, and in our eighties the likelihood is over 65%. This means that most people who live beyond seventy are going to be dealing with this issue.

Low fiber intake is the cause of
constipation, hemorrhoids and diverticulitis

PREBIOTICS ARE BETTER THAN PROBIOTICS

Your colon is not just an empty tube for poop transport; it is also home to trillions of bacteria that function as an important part of your digestive system. These bacteria, otherwise known as probiotics, evolved right alongside humans for millions of years, learning to perform many metabolic and biological functions that humans cannot do on their own. The number of probiotic cells in your body right now outnumbers your human cells by almost 10 to 1, meaning that if we just went by cell count you'd be only 10% human and 90% bacteria. Every year we learn more about the synergistic effects of our probiotics. Probiotics digest fiber and other substances in our diet, and in return they generate antioxidants, provide our colon cells with food to function properly, and ward off infectious disease-causing bacteria. Probiotics also play a role in preventing many conditions, including heart disease, cancer, and obesity, among others.

Probiotics are the topic *du jour* in health circles lately. The number of research articles published on probiotics doubles about every five years, and you can now find probiotic supplements gracing the shelves of your local drugstore and supermarket. But taking probiotic supplements, which actually contain the bacteria themselves, doesn't address the root problem here. You started out your life with plenty of probiotics, so why do you suddenly need more of them? Could it be that you just aren't taking care of the ones you already have?

Rather than pop bacteria-laden pills to try to replenish dwindling supplies of pro-biotics, you could start feeding the ones you do have. It's like when you forgot to feed your goldfish back in grade school so your mom had to keep buying new ones and swapping them out when you weren't looking. Buying a new goldfish is one answer, but then again you could always just start feeding the darn thing and save yourself a trip to the pet store every week.

Fiber is a prebiotic, which is a fancy way of saying "bacteria-food." Since we can't digest fiber, it makes its way all the way down to our colon intact, along with any other bits of food trapped in its matrix. Consequently, fiber is the ideal food source for our healthy bacteria, which have no problem breaking down the bonds that hold fiber molecules together. Without the fiber, there is little for our healthy bacteria to eat after we're done with our meal. Just like man's best friend gnawing on a bone, what we regard as table scraps, they look forward to as a culinary delight.

Fiber promotes the health of good bacteria,
meaning you won't need to take probiotic supplements

YOU SCRATCH MY BACK AND I'LL SCRATCH YOURS

Probiotics don't waste any time helping us out. As soon as they get that first dose of fiber, they start chowing down, and just like us, they have waste products left over after digestion. Good thing for us bacteria waste products happen to be food for our colon cells (see the whole circle of life starting to form before your eyes). Our food waste goes to feed bacteria; their waste goes to feed our colon cells. When bacteria ferment fiber they excrete short-chain fatty acids that are then used as energy by cells in the colon wall, enhancing their ability to function optimally. Since colon cells turn over very quickly, lasting only a few days at most, they need a ready source of fuel. Rather than try to get nutrients from our bloodstream, colon cells find it easier to just draw fuel right from the colon in the form of these short-chain fatty acids, at least when they're available. Not enough fiber means not enough short-chain fatty acids and not enough fuel for our colon cells, meaning they don't function so well.

This might account for some of the colon cancer-preventing effects of fiber. A four-year study showed that patients with higher numbers of **lactobacillus** had reduced recurrence of precancerous colon polyps. Another study showed that patients with colon cancer who were given probiotic supplements of **lactobacillus** and **bifidobacterium** had reductions in a number of cancer markers, including less DNA damage and a reduction in the proliferation of colon epithelial cells. The evidence is mounting that promoting good bacteria is one important way that fiber helps reduce the risk of colon cancer.

Probiotics are also partly responsible for the beneficial effects of the antioxidants we will cover in the next chapter. Antioxidants in soybeans, red wine, tea, and chocolate are partly metabolized by intestinal bacteria into their active compounds that are reabsorbed farther down in the colon. The more probiotics we have, the more antioxidants we can absorb.

Bacterial fermentation also generates one other, less pleasant, byproduct—gas. This alone is enough for most people to try to minimize their dietary fiber intake. Fortunately, there is a fix. Instead of drastically increasing your fiber intake, work your way up slowly. Your body will adapt over time to the increase in fiber, with minimal gas and bloating. Once you get used to the fiber your digestive tract will come back to a normal, healthier, harmony.

WE'RE NOT THE TIGERS WE THINK WE ARE

The bottom line is that your colon (along with the rest of your body) is simply not built for a low-fiber, meat-centric diet. Going back, way back, we evolved from a long line of primates that ate nothing but fruits, veggies, and the occasional insect. Our bodies, and specifically our digestive tracts, are highly adapted to this diet. This doesn't mean that you have to put down your steak knife and start eating ants instead. But it was only in the past million or two years that we started adding meat to our diet, and it was even more recently that we decided that it would be fun to strip all the fiber out of the rest of our diet. Our colons have simply not had time to catch up.

Comparing our digestive system to that of a pure carnivore gives us some perspective on what it takes to live on a high-meat diet. Beyond just sharp fangs and long claws, carnivores have much shorter digestive tracts than do plant-eating creatures. This is possible because meat is a concentrated source of calories. It takes a lot longer to extract 1,000 calories from green leaves than it does from a ½ pound steak. Consequently, a carnivore's intestinal tract is typically half as short as that of a human. With a short digestive tract, a carnivore can readily extract what it needs from its meal and get rid of the waste before it has time to do any harm. For example, a polar bear can digest an entire seal carcass (which has zero fiber) in less than 24 hours. In comparison, a human would need over 60 hours to digest a low- or no-fiber diet. Polar bears are built for meat—their digestive tract doesn't get slowed down on a low-fiber diet at all. Unfortunately, ours does, and we end up paying the price for it.

HUNTER-GATHERER, NOT HUNTER-HUNTER

Our hunter-gatherer ancestors had enviable lives, at least on the surface (forget for a moment the fact that they rarely lived to see thirty). They hunted big game, sat around campfires, and played games all day. Sounds like a great vacation to me, much less a day job. Any man can identify with the macho image of the caveman-as-hunter. Primal, majestic, and only half of the story.

We weren't just hunters; we were hunter-gatherers. The "gathering" part of hunting-gathering was probably a big part of daily life back in the olden days. Experts today estimate that meat made up anywhere from 35% to 55% of daily caloric intake, meaning that anywhere from half to two-thirds of their calories came from plant sources rich in fiber. When you take away all the processed carbs and other empty calories in the Western diet you can actually cram in quite a few grams of fiber in a day and still get plenty of meat. Historical clues support this premise. Analysis of coproliths from just 10,000 years ago suggests that our hunter-gatherer ancestors had as much as 130 grams of fiber daily, way more than we get today. (For those who are curious, a coprolith is fossilized poop. That's right—you've finally found that dream job that your guidance counselor kept secret from you all those years ago: the study of poop fossils.)

It takes a lot to get to 130 grams of fiber. One way to do it would be to have 50 servings of kale or broccoli. Or 48 tablespoons of a fiber supplement. Or 12 handfuls of almonds. These numbers sound crazy but let's put it into context. For one thing, 50 servings of kale sounds like an insane amount of vegetables, but it only adds up to about 1,300 calories, about the equivalent of a Big Mac or a typical pasta dinner at Macaroni Grill. With a 2,500 calorie per day diet, you'd still have plenty of room for more food even after scarfing down your 50th serving of kale. Our ancestors weren't trapped behind a desk all day, so they likely burned even more calories than we do today, leaving them a great deal more room in the diet for all that hunting.

If this sounds impossible, consider the fact that people who live off the land today still consume amounts of fiber approaching ancestral levels. Studies of rural African tribes suggest that their typical fiber intake is in the order of 70–90 grams of fiber daily—not quite the levels of our ancestors but pretty darn close. One reason for the slight decline in fiber intake might be that there are very few true hunter-gatherers left today. Most indigenous tribes have adopted at least some level of agriculture, which you would expect to lead them slowly away from roughage.

These levels of fiber also happen to be roughly equivalent to the amount studied in many trials of cholesterol or blood sugar lowering. For example, in one of the cholesterol-lowering trials mentioned earlier, the high-dose fiber group got a whopping 80 grams of fiber daily. Adding just a little fiber won't move the needle on your cholesterol, but when you get to prehistoric fiber levels, all of a sudden your numbers turn right around. This would explain why many of my patients who think they are getting enough fiber still don't see results the way they should. It also lends credibility to the premise that heart disease and cancer are the consequence of our leaving our natural habitat—if we go back to our natural levels of fiber intake, these diseases practically vanish.

MISSING THE MARK

So if hunter-gatherers should be getting 80+ grams of fiber daily, how close are we getting? Let's start with the recommended daily targets today. The National Cholesterol Education Program recommends that we get at least 30 grams of fiber daily. The government gives us a Recommended Daily Allowance of 38 grams of fiber for men and 25 grams for women. Clearly these targets are far short of what our ancestors got; in fact, cavemen probably flew past the RDA by the time breakfast was over.

So even if we were able to reach these goals we'd still be only about halfway to the minimum hunter-gatherer fiber intake. The bad news is we can't even get that right. A study of over 23,000 Americans showed that we average only 16 grams of fiber daily, which is less than half the RDA for a grown man. Even worse, less than 10% of those studied got to 30 grams of fiber, which *still* is short of the goal. You can start to see now why colonoscopies have become a *de rigueur* part of getting older.

Daily American fiber intake: **Daily hunter-gatherer fiber intake:**

15 grams   130 grams

Now let's consider why none of us get enough fiber. It starts with that way-too-vague definition of what constitutes a healthy diet. A typical "healthy" day might include yogurt or cereal for breakfast, a sandwich for lunch, and then meat, rice, and a side of veggies for dinner. You might even throw in a salad a few days a week. Even if you had whole grain bread and high-fiber cereal, you would still only be getting about 15 to 20 grams of fiber at most, and probably as few as 5 grams of fiber on your off days. Either way, there's no way this diet comes anywhere close to 40 grams of fiber daily.

But what about that high-fiber breakfast bar? Supermarket shelves are stocked with packaged food claiming to be high in fiber. Grab that fiber bar every day and you can comfortably say that you are doing your best to get your fiber. Unfortunately, "high-fiber" is a relative term. According to the FDA, in order to claim that a product is "high-fiber" it must contain 10–20% of the recommended daily allowance. Put another way, the typical high-fiber snack probably contains only 3–4 grams of fiber, which is only one-tenth of the way to your daily *minimum* target. So having one fiber bar daily doesn't justify that warm fuzzy feeling—you'll need another nine bars before you can rest on your laurels.

Fiber supplements can help, but they aren't the whole answer. A tablespoon of psyllium seed husks, the most common fiber supplement, contains 4.5 grams of fiber. Even if you took two tablespoons four times a day, you still wouldn't reach the recommended daily allowance, and it would take another 20 tablespoons to reach hunter-gatherer status. That being said, they are certainly a great adjunct to a diverse hunter-gatherer diet.

THE ANSWER IS B: VEGGIES.

I'll tell you now that the key to getting enough fiber is to drastically rethink the way plants (i.e., veggies) factor into your diet. Most Americans don't get a full serving of veggies until the evening meal, which is way too late to have your first bite of fiber-rich food. You have to get out of the mindset of making vegetables a side dish and put them right in the center of the plate. You've also got to stop putting them off until dinner time and start eating them from the time you wake up to the time you go to bed. It's a modern societal convention to wait until after happy hour to get your first serving of veggies. It's also a societal convention to get diverticulitis and hemorrhoids. So much for convention.

Fiber is only found in plant foods; never in animal products. So the only way to increase your fiber intake is to maximize your intake of vegetables, legumes, nuts, seeds, and fruits (in moderation—remember how much sugar is in modern fruit). If you make these foods a part of every meal then it won't take long to start reaching healthy levels of fiber intake. Along the way you may very well see your cholesterol and blood sugars improve as well.

At the end of this chapter is a table listing the amount of fiber and calories in various plant foods. The table is ranked by the number of calories per gram of fiber. You'll notice that green vegetables have the fewest calories per gram of fiber, while nuts and fruits generally have more. Clearly, you'll get the most fiber by emphasizing the lower-calorie plants simply because you can eat more of them. Expect to start rethinking portion sizes of these vegetables—an entire eggplant has only 140 calories but 16 grams of fiber. Four cups of broccoli have 10 grams of fiber and about 125 calories. Explore ways to make these tasty and you'll find that relatively large portions like these go down very quickly. And start thinking veggies first: "I'll have sautéed broccoli with eggs" is the hunter-gatherer version of "I'll have eggs with some broccoli."

Getting to a hunter-gatherer level of fiber intake won't happen overnight. But over time you can get there and stay there. Try to get in the habit of getting at least 40 grams of fiber daily, which is a reasonable target in modern society. Ideally you'd shoot higher–much higher–but 40 grams is achievable with only a modest amount of effort and puts you head-and-shoulders above your fellow man. If you keep this up you may have something else to talk about over golf other than colon polyps and Lipitor.

You can use online resources like myfitnesspal or calorieking to quantify your daily intake; just log your daily food intake and plug it into the computer at the end of the day to see where you stand. It may seem like a lot of work but after a while you'll be able to estimate your fiber intake without having to look it up each time.

Here's one last tip: try some new flours. Coconut, garbanzo bean, and green pea flours all have a ton of fiber. Start using these flours for some interesting takes on muffins, pancakes, and other quick, ready-made breakfast treats. I've given you some good recipes to start with but enjoy the process of hunting for more.

Challenge #4: Your next Challenge is to start calculating your fiber intake and increase to at least 40 grams of fiber per day. Feel free to use a supplement for up to an additional 10–20 grams of fiber, giving you a more caveman-worthy 60 grams of fiber per day.

Legumes (1 cup cooked)	Fiber (g)	Calories	Cal/g fiber
Green beans	4.0	44	11.0
Kidney beans	16.5	219	13.3
Lentils	15.6	230	1.7
Peas	4.5	67	14.9
Black beans	15.0	227	15.1
Pinto beans	15.4	245	15.9
Garbanzo beans	**12.5**	269	21.5

Seeds (per 10g, about 1 tbsp)	Fiber (g)	Calories	Cal/g fiber
Chia	3.4	49	14.1
Flax	2.7	53	19.6
Sesame	1.2	57	48.6
Sunflower	0.9	58	67.9
Pumpkin	0.6	56	93.2

Nuts (per 40g, or about 30 nuts)	Fiber (g)	Calories	Cal/g fiber
Almond	5.0	232	46.3
Pistachio	4.1	225	54.6
Peanut	3.5	228	65.5
Macadamia	3.4	287	83.5
Walnut	2.7	262	97.6
Cashew	**1.3**	221	167.6

Flours (1/4 cup)	Fiber (g)	Calories	Cal/g fiber
Coconut	10.0	120	12.0
Green Pea	10.7	133	12.5
Garbanzo bean	5.0	110	22.0
Soy	3.0	120	40.0
Almond	3.0	160	53.3

Veggies (1 cup raw)	Fiber (g)	Calories	Cal/g fiber
Radish	1.9	19	10.0
Lettuce (iceberg)	0.9	10	11.1
Kale	2.4	33	13.8
Avodaco	15.6	384	24.6

Veggies (1 cup boiled)	Fiber (g)	Calories	Cal/g fiber
Artichoke hearts	14.4	89	6.2
Spinach	4.3	41	9.5
Cauliflower	1.4	14	10.0
Broccoli	2.6	27	10.4
Asparagus	3.6	40	11.1
Carrots	2.3	27	11.7
Broccoli rabe (one bunch)	12.2	144	11.8
Brussel Sprouts	206	36	13.8
Kale	206	36	13.8
Eggplant	2.5	35	14.0
Zucchini with skin	2.9	38	13.1
Spaghetti squash	2.2	42	19.1
Tomato	1.7	43	25.3
Yam	5.3	158	29.8
Corn	12.1	606	50.1
Veggies (1 large raw)			
Green pepper	2.8	33	11.8
Red pepper	3.4	51	15.0
Avocado	9.2	227	24.7
Onion	3.0	106	35.3
Fruits (1 large raw)			
Asian Pear	9.9	116	11.7
Pear	7.1	131	18.5
Apple (with skin)	5.4	116	21.5
Orange	3.1	69	22.3
Cherries (per cup)	1.6	52	32.5
Banana	4.0	135	33.8
Apply (w/o skin)	2.8	104	37.1
Date	1.6	66	41.3
Grapes (per cup)	1.4	104	74.3
Dried fuits (1 cup loose)			
Apricot	9.5	313	32.9
Prune	12.4	418	33.7
Raisin	5.4	434	80.4

BREAKFAST

Peas for breakfast? Now we're thinking outside the box. If you can handle the thought of green muffins, you can get all the health benefits of legumes from the first meal of the day. You can find the flour at Whole Foods, other specialty shops, or online.

. . . .

GREEN PEA BREAKFAST MUFFINS

4 ripe bananas
¼ cup applesauce

Vanilla extract
2 omega-3 enriched eggs
1 tsp. sodium-free baking soda
1 tsp. cinnamon
¾ cup Bob's Red Mill Green Pea Flour

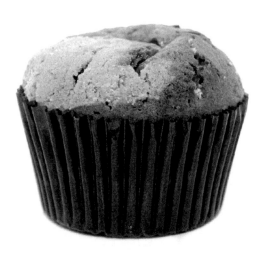

- Preheat oven to 400°F.
- Combine wet and dry ingredients in separate bowls.
- Add wet to dry, combine thoroughly.
- Spoon batter into muffin cups sprayed with olive oil.
- Cook for 15–20 minutes.

YELLOW PEA FLOUR BANANA MUFFINS (ADAPTED FROM CHRIS MARINANGELI)

2 cups yellow pea flour

2 tsp. xanthan gum

1 tsp. cinnamon

½ tsp. nutmeg

2 omega-3 eggs, beaten

¼ cup olive or canola oil

1 cup mashed banana

½ cup water

- Preheat oven to 400°F.
- Combine wet and dry ingredients in separate bowls.
- Add wet to dry, combine thoroughly.
- Spoon batter into muffin cups sprayed with olive oil.
- Cook for 15–20 minutes.

LUNCH, DINNER & SIDES

Wondering what to do with your leftover pea flour from breakfast? Make guacamole, of course! Nothing says healthy like a dip rich in both fiber and monounsaturated fatty acids. Lowering cholesterol never tasted so good.

Green beans are a great, cheap way to get plenty of fiber in your diet. My favorite bean recipe is Loubieh, which can be enjoyed hot but is even better cold or at room temperature. I will often serve it paired with a grilled meat or simply add cooked meat to the pot when done for a one-pot meal that always satisfies.

LEBANESE LOUBIEH

3 pounds green beans

3 medium onions

⅔ cup extra virgin olive oil

1–2 tsp. of Lebanese 7 spice blend*

*equal mixture of allspice, black pepper, white pepper, cinnamon, ground cloves, nutmeg, and coriander

- Rinse the green beans and remove stems.
- Heat oil in large pot on medium.
- Dice onions finely and sauté for about 15–20 minutes.
- Add the green beans and half of the spice mix.
- Mix thoroughly and cover pot, lowering heat to simmer.

- Cook for about 50-60 minutes, stirring every 10 minutes. The beans will be quite dark when done.
- Remove from heat and mix in remaining spices.
- Serve hot or cold, as an entrée or side. Goes well with any grilled meats.

GREEN PEA GUACAMOLE (ADAPTED FROM THE WEBSITE OF BOB'S RED MILL)

2 large mashed avocados

2 tbsp. green pea flour

½ cup water

4 tsp. lemon juice

¼ tsp. chili powder

1 medium diced tomato

1 chopped onion

- Combine water and flour in saucepan and bring to boil. Reduce heat and cook for 3 minutes. Remove from heat.
- Allow to cool, and then add remaining ingredients.

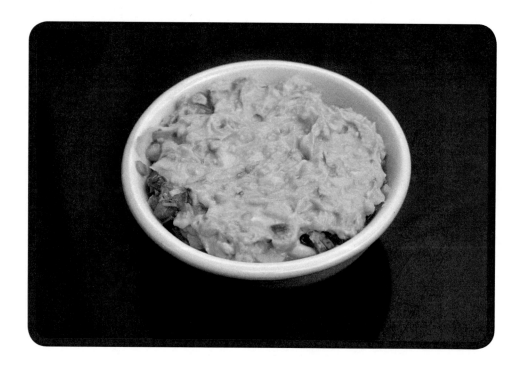

WHITE BEAN AND FENNEL PURÉE

1 can white beans, drained and rinsed
1 onion diced
1 bulb fennel, thinly sliced

1 clove garlic
Olive oil

- Sauté onions until translucent, then add garlic.
- Cook until fragrant.
- Add sliced fennel and cook until soft. Add white beans and cook until heated.
- Place mixture in food processor and puree until smooth.

GREEN PEA SOUP (ADAPTED FROM THE WEBSITE OF BOB'S RED MILL)

1 tbsp. green pea flour
2 cups hot water

2 tsp. salt-free seasoning

- Heat water in saucepan to boil.
- Mix in flour and seasoning, cook for 2 minutes stirring occasionally.

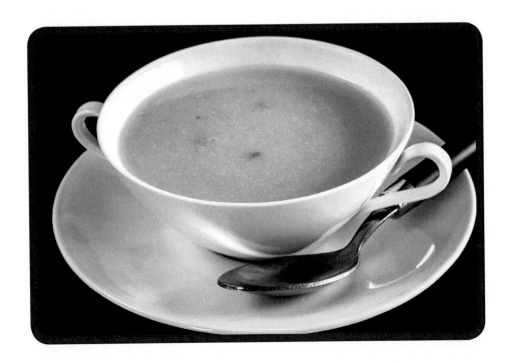

ALMOND GREEN BEANS

1–2 pounds green beans
½ cup slivered almonds

2–4 cloves garlic, minced
Olive oil

- Boil green beans for 5 minutes.
- Drain and return pan to heat.
- Sauté almonds and minced garlic in oil.
- Add beans and toss to coat.

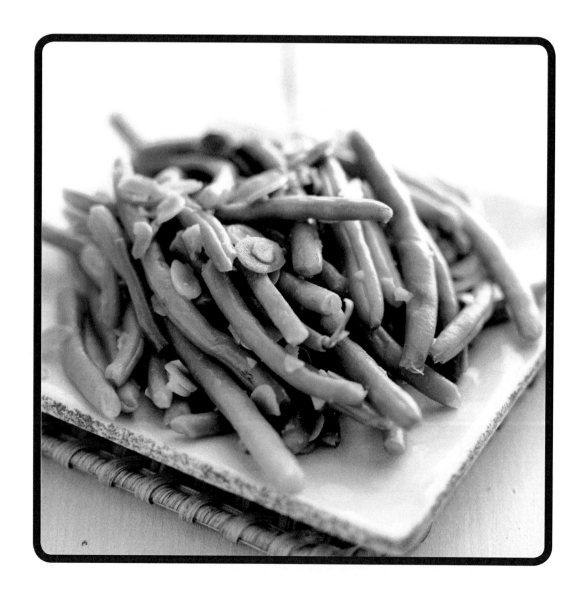

OVEN-ROASTED GREEN BEAN "FRENCH FRIES"

1–2 pounds green beans, trimmed
2 tbsp. extra virgin olive oil

Freshly ground black pepper

- Heat oven to 425°F.
- Toss beans with oil and spread on lined baking sheet.
- Roast for 12–15 minutes, stirring halfway through to cook evenly.
- Can serve in a cup as finger food or as a side.

- Other beans tend to be higher in carbohydrates than green beans or peas, but they have plenty of fiber and a low-glycemic index. Enjoy them but not at the expense of their green cousins.

SAUTÉED ARTICHOKES WITH GARLIC, SHALLOTS, AND SWEET VERMOUTH (ADAPTED FROM JENNIE'S KITCHEN)

1 bag frozen artichoke hearts
1 tbsp. coconut oil or olive oil
1 shallot, thinly sliced

1 clove garlic, thinly sliced
2 tbsp. sweet vermouth
Chopped parsley

- Place artichokes in skillet and cover with water.
- Bring to a boil, cover, and reduce to a simmer. Cook about 10–15 minutes until artichokes are tender.
- Drain artichokes and set aside.
- Clean skillet and place back over medium heat.
- Sauté garlic and shallot for 1–2 minutes. Add artichoke hearts and stir to mix well.
- Cook for 2 minutes, stirring occasionally. Add vermouth and stir, picking up any browned bits stuck to the pan. Cook for 1 minute.
- Stir in parsley and serve warm.

STEAMED ARTICHOKES

2–3 whole artichokes

2–3 cloves garlic

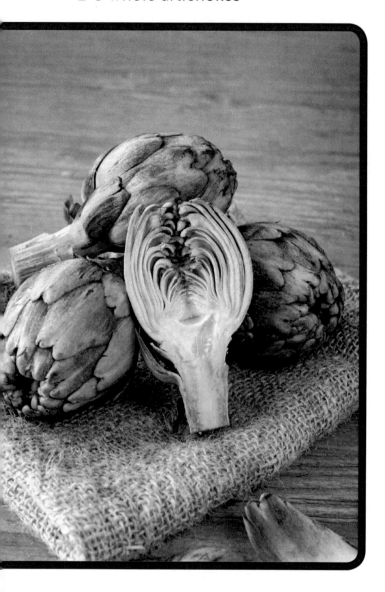

- Bring 1–2 inches of water to boil in a large pot with steamer tray.
- Add garlic to water.
- While water is heating, use shears to trim the points off the artichokes. Then chop about one inch off the top and trim the stem to about 1–2 inches from the bottom.
- Place artichokes in steamer tray and place in pot.
- Cover and steam for 25 minutes.
- Cool and serve. To eat, peel the leaves off the artichoke and bite the soft inner flesh from the inside of each leaf.

WARM ARTICHOKE DIP (ADAPTED FROM JEANETTE'S HEALTHY LIVING)

2 12 oz. bags of frozen artichoke hearts, defrosted
4–6 cloves garlic, minced
2 sprigs of fresh thyme
2 tbsp. plus ¼ cup extra virgin olive oil
Fresh ground pepper to taste

- Preheat oven to 425°F.
- In medium bowl, toss artichoke hearts, garlic, thyme, and 2 tbsp. olive oil. Transfer to foil-lined baking sheet.
- Bake 15–20 minutes uncovered, until garlic is cooked through.
- Remove vegetables from oven and strip thyme leaves from stems, mixing leaves in with vegetables.
- Add vegetables to food processor and blend until smooth, adding olive oil to desired consistency. Season to taste.

Ted B., age 55

When I first met Dr. Dave I was taking one medication for high blood pressure. I didn't think I was doing too badly, but I definitely didn't want to be taking any medication if I could help it.

At the time I was working round the clock starting my own business and didn't think I had any time for diet and exercise. My weight had been a problem since high school and I'd become an expert on getting it off. In fact, three times I had lost 50 pounds, and three times I'd gained it all back again. But despite all the yo-yo dieting I still had high blood pressure and my triglycerides were twice as high as the healthy limit.

Dr. Dave convinced me that not only was the blood pressure curable, but that the yo-yo dieting wasn't getting me anywhere. I definitely didn't argue with that. But I wasn't sure if there was any other way.

Dave invited me to work out with him the very next day. I was pretty skeptical that I could handle any kind of vigorous workout—a college injury had left me with a bum leg a long time ago.

Dave insisted that I give it a try and I did. I ran for the first time in probably 20 years. I did squats and lunges, push-ups and sit-ups. I kept at it for months, and my knee held up. Turns out the knee was fine; I'd just never tried to push it the way Dave encouraged me to.

Two months into the workouts and the diet, my triglycerides had dropped by half, I'd lost over 25 pounds, and was able to throw away my blood pressure medication. Now, over a year later, my blood pressure and triglycerides are still in the normal range and my weight has stayed off. Dr. Dave and Clayton Total Health turned my life around and I'm grateful for it.

CHALLENGE #5: ANTIOXIDANTS— NATURE'S REPAIR CREW

NOW THAT YOU'VE MASTERED HEALTHY FATS, SODIUM, AND FIBER, THERE'S ONLY ONE CHALLENGE LEFT. Luckily, we've saved the best for last, since antioxidants are found in some of our favorite foods like berries, chocolate, and red wine. So if you are ready to finish with some fantastic delicacies that may very well save your life, read on.

Saving your life may sound like hyperbole but it's not. Antioxidants are powerful drugs that actually repair aging cells, prevent disease, and slow the aging process. Missing out on these important compounds puts you at risk for any number of diseases, including dreaded conditions like Alzheimer's dementia and cancer. Let's start by understanding what antioxidants do in your body and how they do it.

RADICAL DAMAGE

Antioxidants are the repair and maintenance crew for your body. Our bodies are like engines, taking in oxygen through our lungs and burning sugar, protein, and fat for energy. The "combustion" of these fuels in the presence of oxygen creates pollution for your body the same way your car creates pollution for the air. In our bodies this "pollution" is in the form of free radicals.

Free radicals are molecules that have an unpaired electron. In chemistry (and your body is one great big chemistry set) all molecular bonds are created through shared electrons. Shared electrons are like a magnet holding together atoms in a molecule. These magnet-like paired electron bonds can be strong enough to hold two atoms together, but given enough force they can be yanked apart. Generating energy from food in our diet creates enough force to do just that. In the process of metabolizing food, a hydrogen atom can be ripped off the surface of a molecule of sugar or fat, leaving it with an unpaired electron. The resulting free radical has the equivalent of a huge magnet on one side, eagerly looking for something to stick to.

If a free radical with an unpaired electron bumps into another molecule—a lipid on the cell membrane, or a protein that is essential for an enzyme reaction in the body—it tries to steal an atom of hydrogen from that molecule. Unpaired electrons are powerful forces, easily strong enough to tear an atom of hydrogen off an unsuspecting nearby molecule. Once this happens, the victim molecule stops doing whatever it was doing and starts its own search for another molecule to attack.

This creates a chain reaction of free radicals that are instantaneously formed and destroyed as one free radical begets another, each time returning to its original, normal state after stealing a hydrogen atom from another molecule.

These chain reactions can be incredibly damaging to cells. We don't have too many molecules we don't need—every protein and lipid in our body serves a purpose. Free radicals cause temporary and often permanent damage by disrupting the normal functioning of molecules in our cells. Free radical damage contributes to many of the conditions we commonly attribute to aging. For example, free radicals create cross-links between collagen fibers in tissues, making stiff and brittle what was once soft and flexible. Collagen is in the lens of our eye, our skin, and our joints. Loss of the elasticity of collagen leads to cataracts, wrinkles, and arthritis as we age. Age-related macular degeneration, the most common cause of blindness in people over 50, is caused by oxidation of the retina by ultraviolet radiation. Neurologic disorders such as Alzheimer's and Parkinson's diseases have been linked to nerve damage from oxidation and free radicals. The inflammation in heart disease—covered in an earlier chapter—is triggered by the oxidation of lipids that are deposited in your arterial walls. Oxidative cell damage has even been linked to diabetes. The list goes on and on.

Managing this damage is critical to our survival, especially since we rely on metabolism of food to survive. Antioxidants are the answer. They stand guard ready to stop chain reactions before they can create disease. Antioxidants are unique in that they can give up a hydrogen atom to a free radical without becoming a free radical in the process. They act like a sponge to absorb free radicals and prevent chain reactions from progressing and wreaking havoc in our bodies.

We humans have our own inherent defenses against free radicals. We have enzymes like superoxide dismutase, which grabs free radicals and converts them to harmless oxygen and water. However, our defenses are simply not good enough to last us a lifetime. Enough free radicals creep in over time to destroy our cells and rob us of our health and youth.

In order to maximize our protection from free radicals we are going to need help, and that help is going to come from our diet. Animals don't have any better antioxidant enzymes than we do so eating them is of little help to us. That extra serving of chicken breast just won't do it. Fortunately, plants have more than enough antioxidants to provide the extra defense we need to ward off disease and stall the aging process.

Antioxidants come in many different forms and can be found throughout the plant kingdom. These include vitamins such as A, C, and E, as well as other molecules called "polyphenols." These include resveratrol, found in grapes and red wine, and curcumin found in the Indian spice turmeric. There are tens of thousands of unique chemical compounds found in nature that act as antioxidants. Many have unique applications in preventing disease: for example, vitamin A and its analogues are important for vision, while polyphenols are important for reducing the lipid peroxidation associated with heart disease. In the following pages we'll see what foods are generally highest in antioxidants then focus on a few important classes of antioxidants that have been studied specifically for disease prevention.

The good news is that pretty much every form of plant life has some amount of antioxidants. *The American Journal of Clinical Nutrition* published a study measuring the antioxidant content of over 1,300 foods common to the American diet. This study included many natural and processed foods and gives us a good look at what foods in our pantry and refrigerator have the most power to stop disease.

The following table on the left shows the top foods according to their amount of antioxidants per gram of food, while the table on the right shows the same data ranked according to antioxidants in a typical serving size. The food with the most antioxidants is given a score of 100% and other foods are ranked accordingly.

For example, on the left hand table, one teaspoon of oregano has 32% of the antioxidant content as one teaspoon of cloves. Clearly, pound for pound, the spices have far and away the most antioxidant power—a teaspoon of cloves has 100x more antioxidants than an equivalent amount of flaxseed or plums. Eight of the top ten foods in the left hand table are spices, with only pecans and walnuts being exceptions. Here in the U.S., you'll find salt and pepper on every table, but you won't find salt on this table at all. Substituting out all the salt and replacing it with delicious flavors from cloves, ginger, turmeric, and mustard seed dramatically changes the health content of what you are putting into your body.

Since you probably will never have a quarter pound of cloves or a teaspoon of plums, the second table gives you a good look at what a typical serving of each food contains in raw antioxidant power. Notice that the top foods include not only berries but many other darkly colored foods like coffee, chocolate, red wine, red cabbage, cherries, plums, and prunes. These foods have rich colors, textures, and flavors along with a healthy dose of antioxidant power.

This study has some limitations, not least of which is the exclusion of certain high-antioxidant foods like green tea and goji berries, which are not part of our typical diet; however, it does give you an idea of how many high-antioxidant foods are already around you. The list does not differentiate between different types of antioxidants but groups them all together based on their ability to stop free radicals in a laboratory. Since we aren't using our food to clean the lab floor, we're going to want to dig a little deeper to understand how to get enough of the right antioxidants to prevent common age-related diseases.

With tens of thousands of antioxidants in our diet, no list of "superfoods" is going to be thoroughly comprehensive—there will always be another trendy food being promoted by the media health experts. That being said, if you are going to start focusing on the antioxidant quality of your diet, few experts would argue that the following foods should top your list.

Antioxidant content for *equal* serving size		Antioxidant content by *typical* serving size	
Cloves, ground	100%	Blackberries	100%
Oregano leaf, dried	32%	Walnuts	65%
Ginger, ground	17%	Strawberries	62%
Cinnamon, ground	14%	Artichokes	62%
Turmeric powder	12%	Cranberries	54%
Walnuts	10%	Coffee	51%
Basil leaf, dried	10%	Raspberries	50%
Mustard seed, ground	8%	Pecans	48%
Curry powder	8%	Blueberries	47%
Pecans	8%	Cloves, ground	46%
Baking chocolate	7%	Baking chocolate	44%
Paprika	7%	Cherries	38%
Chili powder	7%	Red wine	38%
Parsley, dried	6%	Prunes	30%
Dark molasses	4%	Dark chocolate	29%
Black pepper	4%		
Artichokes	3%		
Dark chocolate	3%		
Blackberries	3%		
Cranberries	3%		
Raspberries	2%		
Strawberries	2%		
Blueberries	2%		
Red cabbage	2%		
Red wine	2%		
Prunes	2%		
Cherries	1%		
Red peppers	1%		
Pistachios	1%		
Plums	1%		
Kiwi fruit	1%		
Coffee	1%		
Flaxseed, ground	1%		

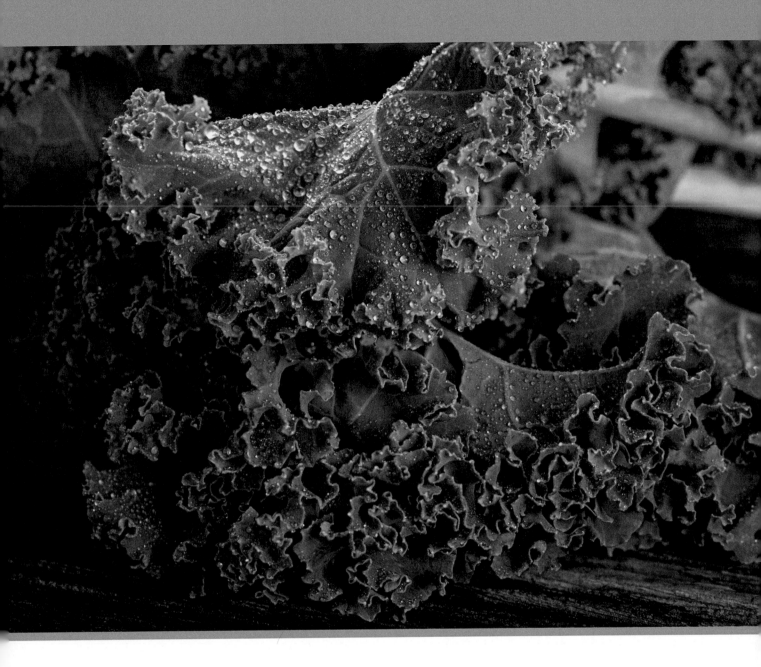

KALE—NOW YOU SEE THE LIGHT

Kale, collard greens, turnip greens, and spinach are all rich in vitamin A derivatives critical for preserving vision. You've heard that kale is good for you, and now it's time to learn why and figure out some ways to include kale and its dark green cousins in your daily routine.

Vitamin A is not just one molecule but represents a family of over 600 similar compounds called "carotenoids." Among them are two that are critical for preserving vision: lutein and zeaxanthin. These antioxidants are absorbed in our diet and concentrated in the retina where they protect the eye from free radical damage. This mechanism is critical to the eye's normal functioning; the eye is constantly exposed to highly focused rays of ultraviolet radiation from the sun, and consequently is the organ most vulnerable to free radical damage. Lutein and zeaxanthin are concentrated in what is called the macular pigment, and when this pigment is depleted blindness occurs.

In addition to being antioxidants, lutein and zeaxanthin actually filter light before it hits the retina, giving us a second layer of protection from the sun's rays. Maintaining adequate levels of lutein and zeaxanthin is our best defense against macular degeneration: a study published in *The Journal of the American Medical Association* showed that people with the highest dietary intake of carotenoids had the lowest risk of developing macular degeneration. Interestingly, taking individual antioxidants other than lutein and zeaxanthin (such as vitamins E or C) had little to no effect on the risk of blindness, while eating vegetables rich in lutein and zeaxanthin, like spinach or collard greens, had the strongest effect, with more than 40% lower likelihood of going blind. Studies suggest that lutein and zeaxanthin taken as supplements have an effect similar to that of dietary sources.

Lutein and zeaxanthin are found in green leafy vegetables such as kale, spinach, collard greens, turnip greens, peas, broccoli, green beans, and lettuce. Other sources of Vitamin A include most brightly colored foods such as butternut squash, carrots, peppers, sweet potatoes, dried apricots, and goji berries.

Lutein and xeazanthin in kale, spinach,
and collard greens prevent age-related blindness

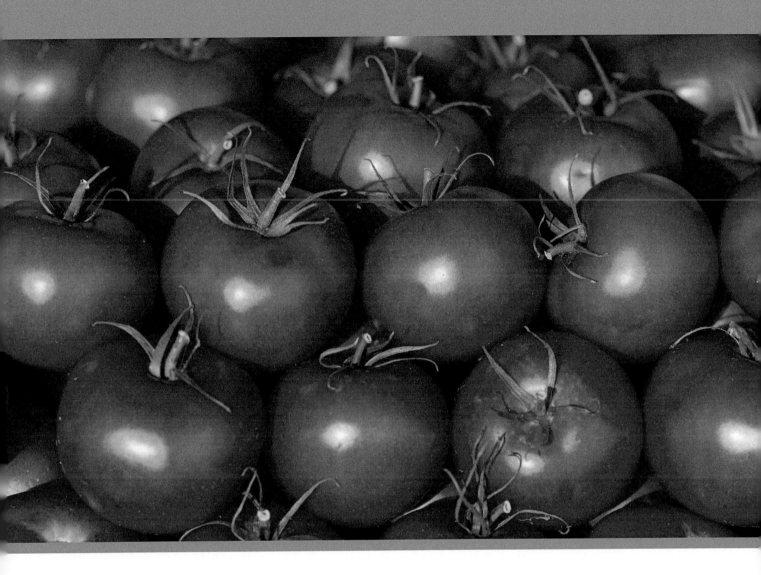

TOMATOES

Tomatoes are a rich source of another carotenoid and powerful antioxidant: lycopene. Like lutein and zeaxanthin, lycopene appears to have tissue-specific effects. Lycopene has been shown to have a protective effect most notably against heart disease and prostate cancer, although studies suggest that it may have additional important roles in protecting from other cancers and even dementia. Lycopene supplementation in the diet can reduce LDL cholesterol and reduce lipid peroxidation, resulting in a reduced risk of heart disease. Tomatoes are probably a significant contributor to the lower risk of heart disease in Mediterranean cultures.

Studies have also shown that there is an inverse association between tomato intake and prostate cancer, making this particularly relevant for men over 50. An analysis of studies on tomato intake demonstrated a 20% reduction in risk of prostate cancer, with one study demonstrating a 40% reduction in risk. Lycopene has also been associated with a lower risk of breast, colon, and lung cancers as well.

Increasing your intake of tomatoes is an important part of the Mediterranean diet and clearly important for decreasing your risk of heart disease. Lycopene is found in most red fruits and vegetables, including papaya, grapefruit, and watermelon in addition to tomatoes. However, over 70% of the lycopene we ingest generally comes from tomatoes and tomato products. This may be because lycopene is actually more readily available from processed compared to raw tomatoes. Crushing and cooking the tomato releases the lycopene so that it can be better absorbed. Tomato paste, tomato sauce, and even ketchup are all sources of lycopene. Lycopene is also better absorbed when it is paired with fat, so cooking with olive oil actually enhances its effectiveness.

The protective effects of lycopene can be achieved by having two or more servings of tomato sauce or its equivalent per week.

Tomatoes are rich in lycopene and are associated with a lower risk of cancer and heart disease. Cooking tomatoes in olive oil releases the lycopene for better absorption.

GREEN TEA

The green tea plant, *Camellia sinensis*, is one of the most potent sources of antioxidants known to man and one of the most studied antioxidant foods in existence—a search of the National Institutes of Health database for "green tea" and "antioxidant" yields over 2,600 results, compared to only 384 results for chocolate. Not only has green tea been extensively researched but the results are remarkable. Consumption of green tea has been demonstrated to improve health by virtually every measure, including reductions of cholesterol and blood pressure, lower risk of heart disease, stroke, and cancer, better immunity from infection by both viruses and bacteria, and even reduction in the risk of osteoporosis.

A review of clinical trials on the effects of green tea on cancer and heart disease published in *The Journal of Clinical Nutrition* demonstrated that green tea consumption had a significant protective effect for prostate cancer (72% reduction in risk) and a modest protective effect for cancers of the breast, esophagus, stomach,

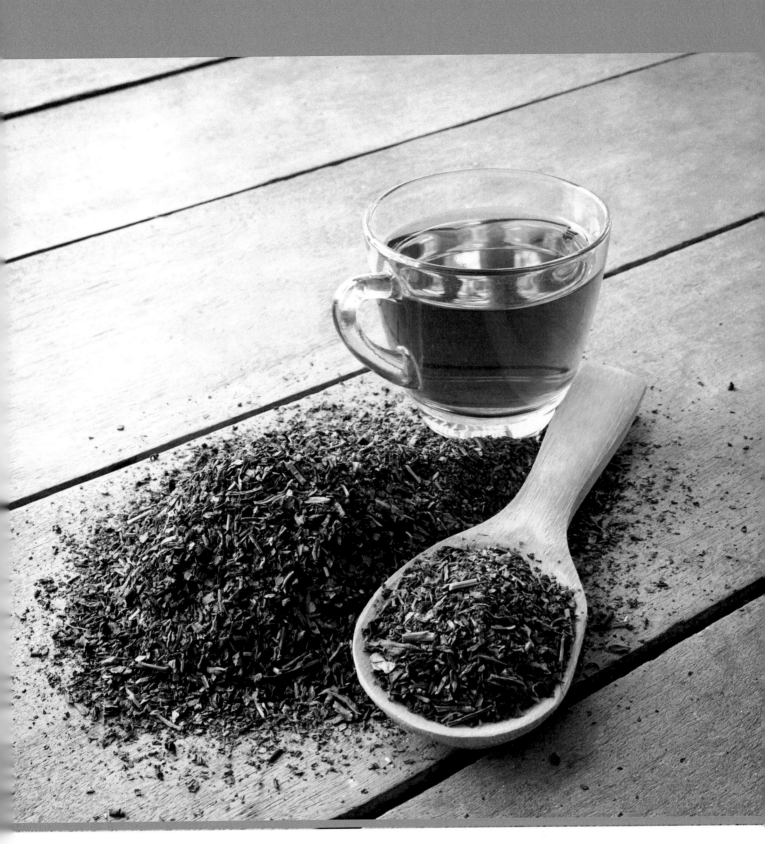

and colon. Another study published in the same journal showed a 28% reduction in risk of heart disease with green tea consumption compared with the consumption of black teas. In this study, it was noted that each additional cup of green tea per day reduced the risk of heart disease by 10% and stroke by over 20%. Makes you want to go down for that coffee—I mean, green tea—break right now, doesn't it?

All teas come from the same tea plant—black, green, oolong, and others are all derived from the leaves of *Camellia sinensis*. The difference between black and green teas is not the plant but how it is processed: if the leaves are prepared raw, the result is green tea; when fermented, the tea becomes black. Green tea preserves most of the antioxidants but has less caffeine—during the fermentation process antioxidants are consumed and the caffeine content increases. Thus, black tea packs more punch to wake you up in the morning but green tea may do a better job of saving your life.

The method of tea preparation also affects its potency. Steeping in hot water releases more antioxidants; the hotter the water and the longer it is steeped, the better. Cold brewed teas still have some antioxidants, just not nearly as many as hot teas. But whether you make your tea hot or cold, you'd better drink it fresh—the longer tea sits, the fewer antioxidants are retained. If you are looking for antioxidant health benefits, store-bought iced teas are probably your worst choice among green teas.

Aside from brewed green tea, there are two other ways of getting your green tea antioxidants if you are unwilling to give up your daily coffee. Extracts of green tea are available as a supplement and generally retain high concentrations of antioxidants. Another option is to use a powdered green tea called "matcha tea," which is a traditional Japanese ceremonial drink. Matcha tea powder can be prepared hot or cold, and makes an excellent addition to smoothies. In fact, this is the type of green tea used for Starbucks-style green tea Frappuccinos. Because matcha tea is consumed whole and not steeped and strained like traditional green tea, it actually retains more antioxidants than even brewed tea. In fact, one study showed that a preparation of matcha tea had over 130 times more antioxidants than a popular brand of green tea, and three times more than the highest amount documented in any brewed green tea in the medical literature.

One cup of green tea a day helps protect against heart disease and cancer, and may reduce blood pressure, cholesterol, and risk of osteoporosis. Hot green tea is better than cold. Matcha powdered tea is the richest source of antioxidants.

SOYBEANS

Unless you are already a vegetarian, it is unlikely that you are getting much soy in your diet. The average American diet includes an average of only one or two servings of *any* beans per week, soy included. This is unfortunate, because soy is one of the most potent disease-fighting foods available; studies suggest that soy may lower the risk of breast and prostate cancers, reduce cholesterol and heart disease risk, improve bone mass, and reduce menopausal symptoms. Men and women alike benefit with no apparent adverse effects, so let's take a moment to learn how soy works this magic and how we can include more in our diets.

The power of soy rests largely in its isoflavones, which are polyphenol antioxidants that happen to also be structurally similar to human estrogen. What makes soybeans special is that it they are the only dietary source of these cancer and heart-disease fighting compounds. Red clover, available as a supplement, is perhaps the only other isoflavone-rich food.

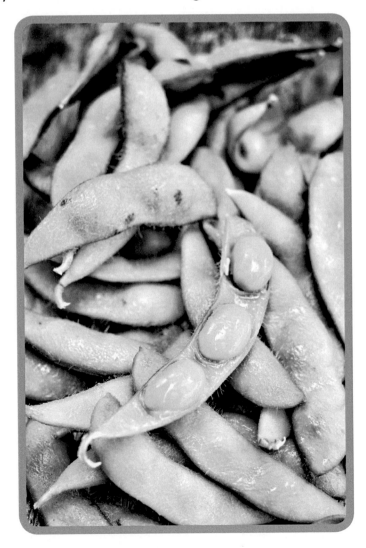

Isoflavones work their cancer-reducing magic in at least two distinct ways. First, isoflavones block an enzyme called tyrosine kinase, which is an important step in cancer proliferation. Tyrosine kinases are the target of many modern cancer drugs, including Sutent and Sprycel. This accounts for at least part of soy's effect of reducing cancer risk.

Second, soy isoflavones bind to receptors for estrogen, keeping your own estrogen molecules from attaching to the same receptors. Your human estrogen works like a light switch, turning on or off receptors for various functions in the body. Isoflavones work more like a dimmer switch, turning on receptors just a little bit, but preventing estrogen from turning them on all the way. This action may account for much of the reduction in risk of prostate and breast cancers, both of which are known to be hormone-dependent. By reducing the "brightness" of the estrogen signal, cancer cells don't have as much stimulation to grow. Studies suggest that men who have high vs. low intake of soy products have up to a 30% reduction in prostate cancer risk. In women the reduction in breast cancer is about the same at around 30%, although there is substantial evidence to suggest that for women the benefit accrues with soy consumption in childhood and adolescence, rather than as an adult. However, soy is not without benefit for adult women; soy consumption may ameliorate menopausal symptoms such as hot flashes. The risk of osteoporosis-associated bone fractures also declines by almost a third among soy enthusiasts.

Soy also works wonders for high cholesterol and heart disease. Soy isoflavones reduce cholesterol, and the soybean is a rich source of plant sterols that block cholesterol absorption in the intestines. In clinical trials, adding soy protein to the diet reduces total and LDL cholesterol by up to 9% and 13%, respectively, with a similar reduction in triglycerides. For most people taking cholesterol medications, this can equate to a 15–20 point drop in total cholesterol. Soy isoflavones have also been shown to dilate arteries, potentially adding another mechanism of fighting vascular disease and improving blood flow to critical organs such as the heart and brain.

How much soy do you need to achieve these goals? The cholesterol- and cancer-fighting isoflavones stay with the soy protein during soybean processing, so it is easiest to think of soy in terms of grams of soy protein. The amount of protein studied in trials ranges up to 60 grams per day, with evidence that as little as 20 g/day may have significant effect. This amount of soy protein generally equates to 25–50 mg of isoflavones. Some studies have shown benefits with much smaller quantities—in some cases as little as one cup of soymilk per day. The take-home message is that some is better than none, although more is probably better than some.

The isoflavone component of soy varies depending on how it is processed: alcohol extraction of the protein removes the isoflavones while water extraction leaves them intact. Thankfully, many supplements will list the amount of isoflavones clearly on the label. Approximately 25–50 mg of isoflavones per day is the range shown to be effective in lowering cholesterol.

Now wait a minute...didn't we just say that soy works like estrogen? So, most guys reading this are probably talking to themselves, saying, "What's this going to do to my manliness and testosterone? No way, Jose...I'll stick with the Lipitor, thank you."

Ok, let's not jump to conclusions. I meticulously perused every available and related study in the National Institutes of Health database to see if soy would cost me my manhood, and here's what I found: soy phytoestrogens in the concentrations needed to lower cholesterol and fight cancer have no effect whatsoever on testosterone levels. In fact, a study of men aged 50–65 showed that results from resistance training actually *improved* with soy protein supplementation. (So real men *can* eat soy.)

Now comes the hard part—getting your daily dose of soy. Options include whole soybeans, tofu, soy milk, and soy protein supplements as well as processed soy foods (e.g., soy burgers, etc.). Soy protein supplements are an easy way to get your soy, but usually come with too much sodium to be strongly recommended. Fermented soy products such as tempeh are more commonly consumed in Asian cultures and may have stronger disease-fighting effects than the tofu or soybeans we think of here in the U.S. At least one cup of soy milk daily or a serving of tofu or tempeh would qualify for a "dose."

When shopping for soy, remember that when soy is processed the healthy isoflavones stay with the protein portion. This means that many soy products, including oil and lecithin, are useless when it comes to the health benefits. In fact, soy oil is rich in omega-6 and therefore should be avoided.

Soy protein in soybeans, tofu, and tempeh reduces cholesterol and lowers cancer risk without reducing testosterone levels in men

---

CURCUMIN

Curcumin is a polyphenol antioxidant found in the Indian spice turmeric, derived from the roots of the *Curcuma longa* plant. Curcumin has been used as a medicinal herb for centuries, purported to cure everything from abdominal bloating to arthritis. Modern studies show that curcumin has multiple effects, including antiviral, antioxidant, and anti-inflammatory activity. In preclinical studies curcumin has inhibited the progression of blood, skin, and colon cancers, reduced the symptoms of certain forms of arthritis, improved wound healing, reduced the progression of vascular disease, and reversed the formation of brain plaques associated with Alzheimer's dementia.

Perhaps most compelling is the data on curcumin for the treatment or prevention of Alzheimer's dementia. The Indo-U.S. Cross National Dementia Study compared rates of dementia among the elderly in a small village in India with those of a rural town in Pennsylvania. The study found that 5% of Pennsylvanians over 70 had dementia, compared to only 1.7% in India. The risk of having dementia in the U.S. appears to be about three times greater than in India. This may be a function of genetics, but diet appears to also play a significant role. Another study of over 1,000 elderly individuals demonstrated that those who ate yellow curry, high in curcumin, less often than once every six months were twice as likely to have dementia as those who ate curry at least once a month. This is consistent with laboratory studies that suggest that curcumin has the ability to actually prevent the beta-amyloid plaques in the brain that are the hallmark of Alzheimer's disease.

The optimal dose of curcumin is unknown, but based on these studies and others, it is likely that curcumin need not be taken in high doses or even daily to have a significant effect. The best-performing subjects in the dementia study above only had curry once a month or more on average. Most studies use anywhere from 500 milligrams to over 3,000 milligrams daily as a curcumin supplement taken in pill form, with higher doses thought effective for the control of blood sugars and improvement in diabetes, among other things.

Turmeric is the yellow curry spice from which curcumin is derived. About 3% of the weight of turmeric is curcumin, so if you are attempting to get 500 milligrams of curcumin, you'll need about 15 grams of turmeric per person, which is equivalent to about a tablespoon. Having done this myself I will tell you that this much curry is an acquired taste, but doable. Another reasonable approach, given the data, would be to either take a supplement or to simply enjoy curry once or twice a month as part of your routine. There are plenty of great curry recipes out there that may help you preserve your brain as well as your body.

Curcumin in turmeric and curry reduces risk of Alzheimer's disease. One tablespoon of turmeric contains a 500 milligram dose of curcumin. Having curry or turmeric at least once a month may be enough to reduce the risk of dementia.

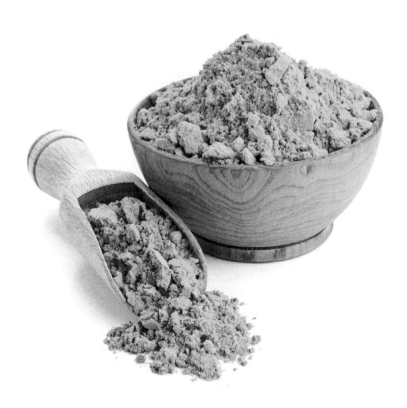

RED WINE

All alcoholic beverages in moderation will raise HDL ("good") cholesterol and reduce heart disease risk; however, red wine's benefits go beyond those of other alcoholic beverages. The reason for this is the antioxidants found in the skin of the red grape, which have been studied for their effect on reducing heart disease and even increasing longevity.

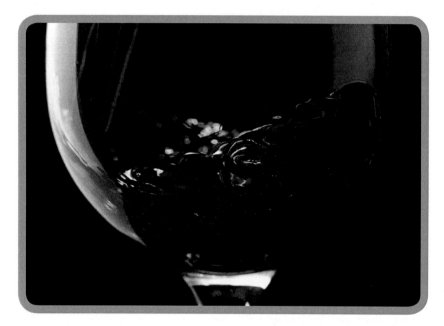

Perhaps the greatest benefit of drinking red wine (other than the obvious social benefits) is its protective effect in heart disease; red wine consumption is one of the reasons that the French tend to get less heart disease than do Americans. The antioxidants in red wine are effective in reducing the oxidation of lipids that causes them to be deposited in our arteries, eventually leading to heart attack and stroke. A study performed in the U.K. showed that blood samples from people drinking one glass of red wine or the equivalent amount of alcohol-free red wine extracts had lower amounts of oxidized LDL cholesterol. The control group, who enjoyed white wine, had greater numbers of oxidized particles in the blood. Red wine is the only alcoholic beverage that has this effect.

But the benefits of red wine don't stop at preventing the oxidation of lipids—red wine actually might trick the body into living longer. Red wine is rich in one antioxidant—resveratrol—that makes your body think that you are eating less, thereby resetting your biological clock and perhaps helping you live longer.

Calorie restriction is perhaps the most well-studied and proven mechanism of extending the useful life of the body. Restricting calories by 30–40%, while maintaining adequate nutrition, extends the lifespan of laboratory animals and protects against diabetes, cardiovascular disease, and cancer. Now that we understand how oxidation takes place it makes sense that reducing calories, and therefore the free radical "pollution" that burning calories creates, would reduce the wear and tear on the body and extend life. Most of the free radical damage in our bodies is a byproduct of metabolizing food; if we decrease the amount of food we ingest, our bodies should last longer.

Despite the benefits of prolonged calorie restriction, maintaining a low-calorie diet is difficult if not impossible. Anyone who has gone on a typical diet can tell you this—most people don't even make it six months, much less a lifetime. This is where resveratrol comes in.

Resveratrol activates an enzyme called "Sirt1," which is partially responsible for the beneficial effects of calorie restriction. By tricking this enzyme into thinking that you are indeed starving (with no effect on your conscious level of hunger) you may be able to achieve the same results. Theoretically, this should work in humans: in animal studies resveratrol does indeed protect against obesity, diabetes, and premature cell death. Research is still inconclusive, but it is nice to know that each sip of red wine may give you more days to enjoy it.

One to two glasses of red wine a day prevents the oxidation of lipids that leads to heart attack and stroke.

CHOCOLATE

It sometimes seems that every day there's another news flash touting the health benefits of chocolate. The notion of chocolate as health food has a "too good to be true" feel to it; however, in this case the good news *is* true. The cocoa bean is a rich source of flavanol-type antioxidants and is one of the most potent antioxidant-rich foods within our reach. Dark chocolate and other cocoa products have been associated with reduced cholesterol, lower blood pressures, improved insulin sensitivity, and a reduction in the risk of heart disease.

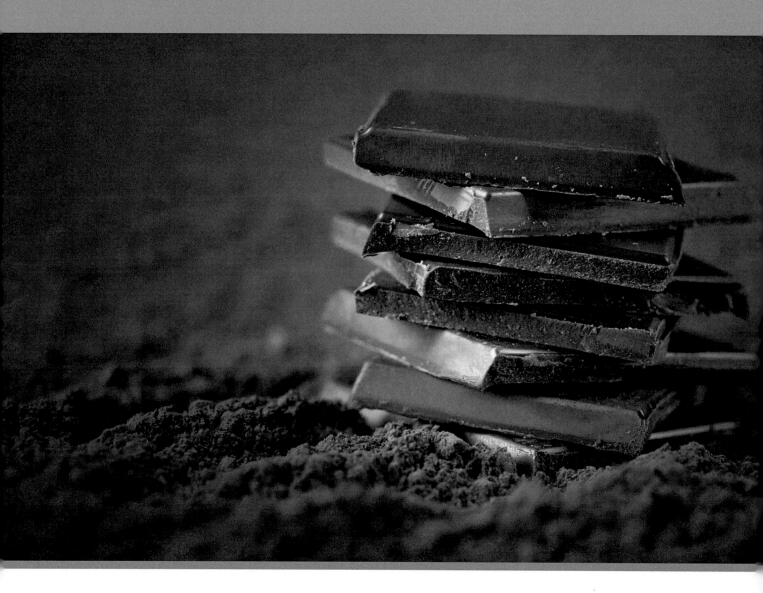

Let's first look at the data on cholesterol. Stearic acid, the primary constituent of cocoa butter, is a saturated fatty acid. Therefore, after our experience learning about healthy and unhealthy fats, we know that chocolate should raise our LDL and total cholesterol levels.

Prepare to be pleasantly surprised. Stearic acid is perhaps the only saturated fat that actually lowers LDL and total cholesterol. A review of trials including almost 1,000 patients showed that enjoying chocolate provided modest improvement in LDL cholesterol while also marginally increasing HDL. Think about that one for a minute: chocolate actually may improve your cholesterol levels. Wow.

Chocolate also may improve your blood pressure; a review of dark chocolate's effects on blood pressure showed that in patients with hypertension (blood pressure 140/80 or above), eating chocolate actually lowered blood pressure by up to 5 points, while there was no effect on patients with normal blood pressure.

Apparently, the effect of the chocolate is even more specific than that of a drug, targeting only those who need it and sparing those who do not.

Another trial confirmed these results, showing that dark chocolate lowered blood pressure (this time by about 4 points), lowered LDL cholesterol by 7.5%, and actually improved insulin sensitivity compared to a control group eating white chocolate. This insulin sensitivity part is important–chocolate ingestion has actually been shown to improve diabetes and prediabetes by improving the body's ability to respond to insulin. A review of over 1,200 patients published in *The American Journal of Clinical Nutrition* showed that dark chocolate actually lowers blood sugar and insulin levels and improves insulin sensitivity.

Cocoa products, specifically cocoa antioxidants, offer improvements in cholesterol, blood pressure, and blood sugars. You would think that would translate to better longevity, and you'd be right. Compared to those who denied their chocoholic tendencies, patients who'd had a previous heart attack and who indulged at least twice a week were 66% less likely to die over an eight-year period. Did longevity ever taste so sweet?

The primary flavanol in cocoa beans is epicatechin, and studies suggest that it takes at least 50–100 mg of epicatechin to get the amazing health benefits of chocolate. Raw cocoa beans, available as cocoa nibs, have the most antioxidant of any cocoa product. Unfortunately, processing the cocoa bean threatens these powerful compounds. Flavanols are bitter to taste, and are generally removed in the process of making chocolate smoother and sweeter. In fact, the smoother and sweeter the chocolate, the fewer flavanols are likely to be there.

So bitter chocolate is better chocolate. The bitterest chocolates are cocoa nibs, unsweetened cocoa powder, and baker's chocolate, all of which have the highest amounts of flavanols among chocolate products. An industry-sponsored study of commercially available chocolate products (excluding nibs) found that cocoa had the highest proportion of flavanols, followed by baking chocolate, and dark chocolate. In last place was milk chocolate and chocolate syrup, both of which are essentially devoid of flavanols.

	SERVING SIZE (g)	EPICATECHIN (mg)	FLAVANOLS (mg)
Cocoa powder	10	18.5	227.3
Baking chocolate	15	17.1	226.5
Dark chocolate	40	13.5	145.8
Semi-sweet chips	15	7.3	73.4
Milk chocolate	40	4.0	27.4
Chocolate syrup	39	2.9	25.8

If you have room for a few hundred extra calories in the diet, you can reach for the dark chocolate. If not, you'd better stick to cocoa powder or cocoa nibs. Two tablespoons of cocoa contains about 227 mg of flavanols, just over 18 mg of epicatechin, and 12 calories. To get the amount of flavanols studied in clinical trials you'd need about six tablespoons per day for about 72 calories. The equivalent amount of baking chocolate would cost you 450 calories. Puts chocolate as a health food in perspective, doesn't it?

Unsweetened cocoa has the most antioxidants with the fewest calories, followed by baker's chocolate and dark chocolate (>60% cocoa solids) Two servings of chocolate per week may lower your risk of heart attack or stroke

So which one to buy? Plain old Hershey cocoa has plenty of flavanols and is one of the cheaper options available—in fact, they sponsored the above study on the flavanol content of chocolates. Supplements are also available to offer essentially calorie-free access to the health benefits of chocolate. Two brands to look for are CocoaWell and CocoaVia, both available on Amazon or at specialty stores. Lastly, you can go *au naturel* and buy raw cacao nibs, which are completely unprocessed and contain the highest amounts of flavanols. Most specialty stores like Whole Foods carry these as well. Bon appétit!

Challenge #5: For the next two weeks move your antioxidants to the center of the table. Enjoy one high-antioxidant food with each meal of the day. Choose among varied spices, teas, fruits and vegetables, berries, and more. Top it off with a dark chocolate dessert for good measure, but keep your eye on the calories!

KALE RECIPES

SAUTÉED KALE (ADAPTED FROM BOBBY FLAY)

1½ pounds kale, chopped coarsely

2 tbsp. olive oil

2 cloves garlic, sliced thinly

½ cup water

2 tbsp. red wine vinegar

- Heat oil in saucepan over medium heat.
- Add garlic, cook until soft.
- Add kale and water, turn heat to high and cover for 5 minutes.
- Remove cover and cook, stirring frequently until water has evaporated.
- Remove to plate, toss with vinegar, and serve.
- For a variant on this recipe, try adding chopped mushrooms with the garlic.

BUTTER BEANS, KALE, AND EGGS (ADAPTED FROM SERIOUSEATS.COM)

1 pound butter beans (large lima beans)

3–4 oz. pork loin

2 quarts no-sodium homemade or canned chicken broth

2 bay leaves

4 thyme sprigs

1 whole onion, split in half

1 medium carrot

1 rib celery

1 28 oz. can whole tomatoes packed in juice, roughly chopped

4 cups roughly chopped kale or curly spinach leaves

2–4 hard-boiled eggs

2 tbsp. extra virgin olive oil

Freshly ground black pepper

- Cover beans with 2 quarts cold water.
- Stir once to combine then set aside at room temperature for at least 8 hours.
- Drain and rinse beans and add to a large saucepan.
- Add pork, chicken broth, bay leaves, thyme, onion, carrot, and celery.
- Bring to a boil over high heat, reduce to a simmer, and cook until beans are completely tender, about 1 hour, topping up with water as necessary (beans should be just poking through the top surface).
- Discard bay leaves, thyme sprigs, onion, carrot, and celery. Remove pork and discard if desired or chop up and add back to pot.
- Add tomatoes and kale to pot, bring to a simmer, and cook, gently stirring occasionally with a wooden spoon until thickened and stew-like, about 20 minutes longer.
- Season to taste with pepper and serve topped with hard-boiled eggs and a drizzle of extra virgin olive oil.

CURRY (CURCUMIN) RECIPES

OKRA WITH YELLOW CURRY

1 pound okra, sliced into ¼ inch rounds
1 tbsp. olive oil
1 tsp. whole cumin seeds
1 tbsp. turmeric powder
½ tsp. chickpea flour

- Microwave okra on high for 3 minutes.
- Heat olive oil in large skillet over medium heat.
- Add cumin and stir constantly until golden brown.
- Stir in turmeric and cook for another 1–2 minutes, stirring constantly.
- Stir in chickpea flour followed by okra.
- Cook together for 2 minutes.
- Remove from heat and serve immediately.

CURRY CHICKEN

3 tbsp. olive oil

1 small onion, chopped

2 cloves garlic, minced

3 tbsp. curry powder or turmeric powder

1 tsp. ground cinnamon

1 tsp. paprika

1 bay leaf

½ tsp. grated fresh ginger root or dried ginger

2 skinless, boneless chicken breast halves cut into bite-size pieces

1 tbsp. salt-free tomato paste

1 cup coconut milk

½ tsp. cayenne pepper

- Heat olive oil in a skillet over medium heat.
- Add curry powder, cinnamon, paprika, and cayenne pepper and stir for 2 minutes.
- Add bay leaf, followed by garlic and onion.
- Stir until lightly browned.
- Add chicken pieces, tomato paste, and coconut milk.
- Bring to a boil, reduce heat, and simmer for 20 to 25 minutes, until chicken is cooked through and tender.

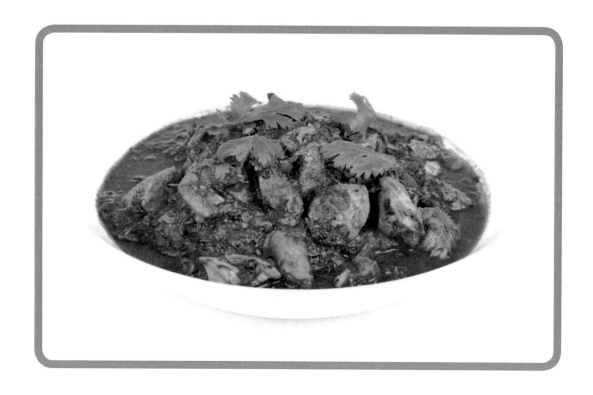

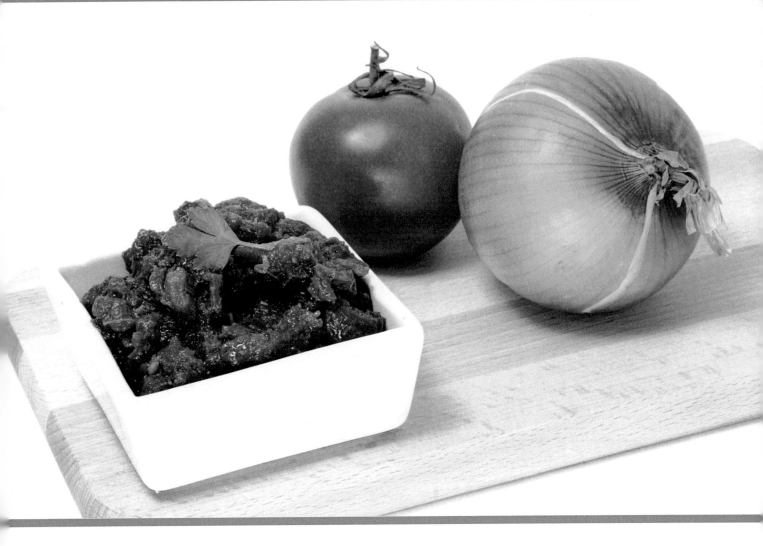

TOMATO RECIPES

SOFRITO

2 medium green peppers
2 sweet red peppers
2 large tomatoes
2 medium onions

1 head of garlic
1 bunch cilantro leaves
½ bunch parsley leaves

- Peel garlic and onions, remove seeds from peppers.
- Chop vegetables and add to food processor. Pulse until chopped finely.
- Heat olive oil in large pot over medium heat.
- Sauté for 20–30 minutes until thickened and reduced.
- Store in a glass, airtight container to preserve antioxidants.

EASY SOFRITO

3-4 hothouse tomatoes chopped into 1-inch cubes

4-5 cloves of garlic, peeled and chopped roughly

1 large onion, diced

Olive oil

Mrs. Dash spice blend

- Heat a generous amount of olive oil over medium heat.
- Add tomatoes, onions, garlic cloves, and spices.
- Cover and simmer until tomatoes and garlic are soft, about 15 minutes.
- Serve as a side or main dish.

Sofrito is an easy way to start lending a Mediterranean flavor to your home-cooked meals. It can be stored for several days and used to top meats or vegetables in place of a store-bought tomato sauce.

EASY SAUTÉED TOMATOES

2-3 large tomatoes

3 tbsp. olive oil

Pepper to taste

- Chop tomatoes roughly into 1-inch cubes.
- Sauté over medium heat until soft.
- Season and serve.

MAMA'S HOMEMADE TOMATO SAUCE

¼ cup olive oil

1 Spanish onion, diced

4 cloves garlic, peeled

3 tbsp. fresh thyme or 2 tbsp. dried

½ carrot, grated

4 pounds of tomatoes, peeled and crushed

- Cook onion and garlic over medium heat for 8-10 minutes.
- Add thyme and carrot, simmer for another 5 minutes.
- Add tomatoes and thyme.
- Simmer for about 30 minutes to reduce.

SUMMER GAZPACHO

6 ripe tomatoes
½ large cucumber
1 green pepper
2 cloves garlic

1 cup water
⅓ cup extra virgin olive oil
Juice of one lime

- Chop all vegetables and combine with liquid ingredients in food processor.
- Puree until smooth. Pour and serve.

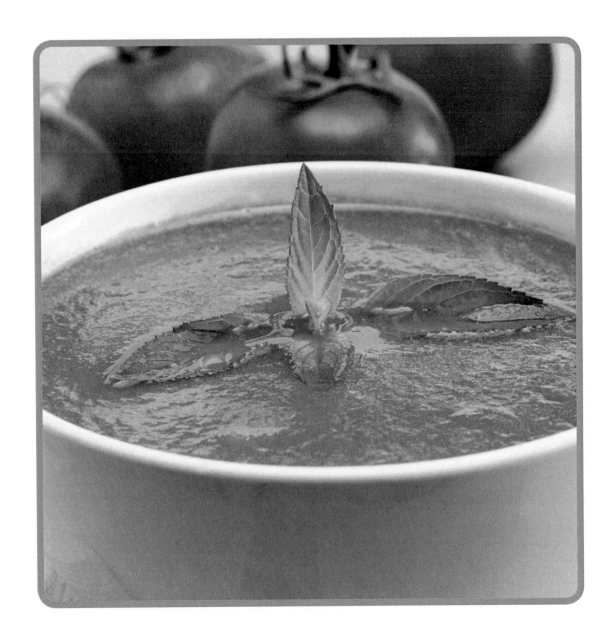

MARINATED TOMATOES

3 tbsp. chopped parsley
3-4 tsp. Mrs. Dash
¾ tsp. dried thyme
¾ cup olive oil

2-3 green onions, chopped
4-6 large hothouse tomatoes, each cut into 6 wedges

- In a mixing bowl thoroughly combine all ingredients except tomatoes.
- Add tomatoes to a dish or bag for marinating (Ziploc plastic bags work well). Pour marinade over and let rest at room temperature for up to 2-3 hours.

SOY RECIPES

SUPER EASY TOFU TACOS

1-2 pounds of extra firm tofu (each pound of tofu when drained will yield about ⅓ to ½ pound of tofu)
1 head of iceberg lettuce

Salsa fresca (finely chopped tomatoes, onions, garlic, and cilantro)
Guacamole or avocado
Soy cheese (shredded mock cheddar)
One packet taco seasoning

- Take a block or two of extra firm tofu and crumble it into cheese cloth.
- Squeeze vigorously to release as much moisture as possible. Wringing the tofu is effective. The drier it is, the better the texture when cooked.
- Sauté in a little olive oil, as you would ground beef for tacos.
- Cook for about 3-5 minutes. The tofu will brown slightly.
- Add taco seasoning to taste and water according to package instructions.
- Stir to mix.
- Wash lettuce and carefully separate into individual whole leaves.
- Wrap taco meat, guacamole, and salsa fresca in lettuce leaves and serve immediately.

SPICY TOFU AND BROCCOLI RABE

For the tofu:

3 tbsp. freshly squeezed lemon juice
2 tbsp. freshly chopped basil leaves
2 tbsp. extra virgin olive oil
1 tbsp. balsamic vinegar

1 tsp. finely grated lemon zest
1 pound firm tofu, rinsed, patted dry
and sliced ½ inch thick

For the broccoli rabe:

2 pounds broccoli rabe, tough stalks
trimmed
4 tbsp. extra virgin olive oil
8 plump cloves garlic

½ tsp. hot red pepper flakes
Freshly milled black pepper
Lemon wedges, for garnish

- Preheat oven to 375°F.
- In a bowl, combine the lemon juice, basil, oil, vinegar, and lemon zest.
- Lay the tofu slices in a baking dish that can hold them in a single snug layer. Pour the marinade over the tofu.
- Bake for 30 minutes, or until the tofu is nearly dry and well browned.
- To make the broccoli rabe, chop the tender stalks and greens into 2-inch pieces and soak them in a large basin of cold water.
- In a heavy, wide sauté pan over medium heat, warm the oil.
- Add the garlic and sauté gently for 3 to 5 minutes, until golden.
- Add the red pepper flakes and tofu and sauté for 1 minute. Scoop the greens from the water and add them to the pan.
- Raise the heat and turn the greens over in the oil with a pair of tongs.
- When the greens begin to simmer, reduce the heat to low and cover. Cook for 10 to 15 minutes, until the greens are tender.
- Season with pepper (no salt!) and serve garnished with the lemon wedges and garlic cloves.

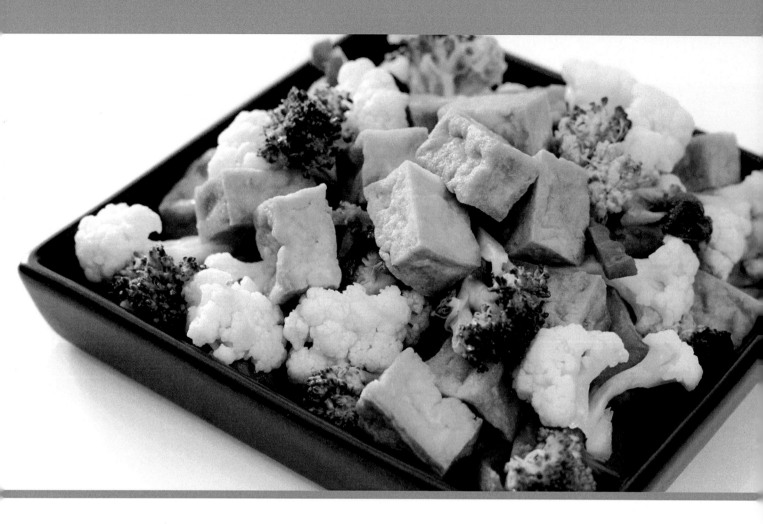

TOFU STIR-FRY

1 block of extra firm tofu
1–2 bags of frozen mixed vegetables
Olive oil

Ginger, sliced scallions, minced garlic to taste

- Stir-fry the vegetables in olive oil until cooked thoroughly.
- Add tofu, heat, and serve.

COCOA & CHOCOLATE RECIPES

DR. DAVE'S FAMOUS AVOCADO CHOCOLATE PUDDING

2–3 avocados
¼ cup unsweetened cocoa powder

2 tbsp. honey
1 tsp. vanilla extract

- Combine ingredients in food processor or mixer.
- Blend until smooth.

COCOA NIB HOT CHOCOLATE (ADAPTED FROM ALTON BROWN ON THE FOOD NETWORK)

1 oz. cocoa nibs

16 oz. soy or almond milk

6 oz. dark chocolate (85% or greater), finely chopped

1 tbsp. honey (optional)

2 oz. water

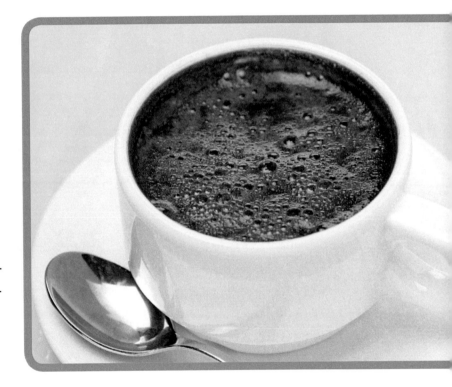

- Pulse the cocoa nibs in coffee grinder until coarsely chopped.
- Place in a 1-quart microwave-safe measuring cup and add the milk. Microwave on high for 3 to 4 minutes or until the milk reaches 160°F. Steep at room temperature for 30 minutes.
- Meanwhile, combine the remaining ingredients in a 1-liter French press. Set aside.
- After steeping, return the nib–milk mixture to the microwave and heat on high for 2 minutes until it simmers or reaches 185°F.
- Strain the hot nib–milk mixture through a fine-mesh strainer into the French press carafe. Set aside for 1 minute, and then stir to combine the chocolate and milk.
- Pump the plunger of the French press 10 to 15 times to froth and aerate. Serve immediately.

TRIPLE CHOCOLATE TRUFFLES (ADAPTED FROM PALEOMG.COM)

7 medjool dates, pitted
1 cup pumpkin seeds
3 tbsp. unsweetened cocoa powder
1 tbsp. honey
1 tsp. vanilla extract

¼ tsp. cinnamon
4–5 oz. 85% dark chocolate or higher, melted
Small dark chocolate chips
1 tbsp. olive oil

- Place a small skillet over medium heat and add your tablespoon of oil.
- Toss in your pumpkin seeds to begin to roast, moving them around often, being sure not to burn them.
- Cook pumpkin seeds for about 3–5 minutes, until they become fragrant and slightly browned.
- Add to food processor and pulse until they are completely broken down into a pumpkin seed meal.
- Add dates and puree until smooth.
- Add cocoa powder, honey, vanilla, and cinnamon and blend thoroughly. The mixture should have the consistency of dough.
- Tear off pieces by hand and roll into balls. Place on parchment paper.
- Separately, use a double boiler or a pan on low heat to melt chocolate. Keep warm for dipping.
- Push a toothpick into each ball of dough and dip it in

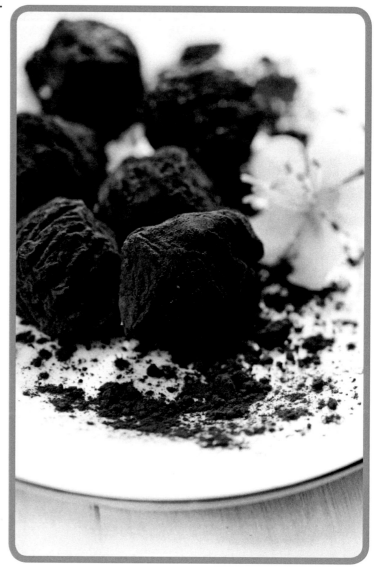

the chocolate, then follow by dipping in chocolate chips. Place on a parchment paper covered plate.

- Place in refrigerator for the chocolate to harden and set.

. . . .

CHOCOLATE MOUSSE (ADAPTED FROM PALEODIETLIFESTYLE.COM)

¼ cup chocolate pieces (> 85%)
½ cup light coconut milk, soy milk, or almond milk
1 tbsp. ground coffee beans

¼ cup water
1 tbsp. vanilla extract
¼ tsp. coffee extract

- Using a skillet or double boiler, melt chocolate over low to medium heat, stirring frequently.
- Add milk, stirring to mix thoroughly.
- Boil water and mix in ground coffee in separate bowl.
- Combine the melted chocolate, coffee mixture, vanilla extract, and flavored extract.
- Separate into serving-size cups and refrigerate for at least 2 to 3 hours until firm.
- Serve cold.

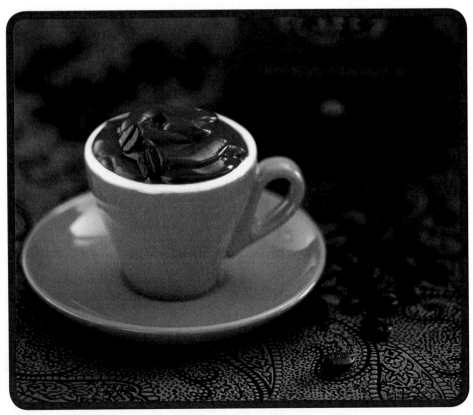

TOFU CHOCOLATE MOUSSE

8–12 oz. dark chocolate (preferably 60–100% cocoa, the higher the better)

24 oz. silken tofu

2 tsp. vanilla extract

4 egg whites

- Melt the chocolate over low heat, stirring often.
- Blend tofu in a food processor.
- Add the vanilla and melted chocolate and blend again, stopping once or twice to scrape down the sides of a bowl with a rubber spatula.
- Beat the egg whites to soft peaks.
- Place the tofu chocolate mixture into a bowl and slowly fold in the egg whites with a rubber spatula.
- Refrigerate for several hours before serving.

This is one of my favorite recipes. It takes minutes to make, is absolutely delicious, and is super healthy.

YOU DID IT!!!!

CONGRATULATIONS! Whether it's been one month, three months, or six months, you've finished all the Challenges. By now you should know more than your own doctor when it comes to nutrition and your health. More than likely you've been able to stride back into the exam room with your head held high and gloat over your success. If you've been following the metrics I laid out upfront, you can be certain that one or more have moved significantly in the right direction. In fact, the only people I've ever seen *not* improve with this plan are the ones who just don't do it. Everyone else sees the benefits, and most of the time the success becomes addictive.

As you go forward you should be thinking about food in a whole new light. Food is a powerful drug that can heal or promote disease, and now you have the ability to see through marketing messages and sound bites to identify the foods that truly do promote good health. Continue to make the right choices and your health will continue to improve.

On the next two pages I've given you a summary of the take-home messages in the book. What always amazes me is that with just a few lessons we've covered the root causes of nearly every major chronic medical problem we face as we get older. Glance down the far right column and you'll see that everything you've ever worried about or talked to your doctor about is probably on that list. It's like I said at the very beginning—five simple rules account for over 70% of chronic disease. These five lessons may very well be all you need to know to reverse disease, get off medications, and add years to your life.

Now that you're an expert you may be tempted to put this book away or lend it to a friend, but I recommend you keep it handy for a reference now and then. We all have days (or weeks) when we slack off for one reason or another. As you come off a slump you'll want to refresh your memory about sodium or healthy fats. You may even want to go through a few of the Challenges again just to get back on top of your commitment to good health.

However you use this book, I congratulate you on your success and wish you your absolute best health—and best life—going forward.

WHAT TO GET	HOW MUCH TO GET	WHERE TO GET IT	WHAT IT DOES	WHAT IT TREATS
Omega-3s	At least 2,000 milligrams	Oily fish: tuna, salmon, halibut, sardines, anchovy Grass-fed or pastured meats Omega-3 enriched eggs Chia, flax seeds	Reduces inflammation	Alzheimer's disease Heart attack and stroke Cardiac death Asthma Arthritis
Fiber	At least 40 grams	Vegetables: artichokes, spinach, cauliflower, broccoli, radish, green pepper Legumes: green beans, lentils	Prevents absorption of toxins and cholesterol Promotes healthy bacteria Improves stool transit	High cholesterol Heart disease Colon and other cancers Constipation Hemorrhoids Diverticulitis
Antioxidants	As much as possible	Vegetables: Kale, spinach, collard greens, sweet potatoes, peppers, and more Soybeans, green tea, cocoa, berries, red wine Spices: cloves, mustard, cinnamon, oregano, basil	Prevents free radical damage Reduces oxidation of lipids	Cancer, Heart attack and stroke Age-related blindness, Wrinkles, Cataracts Arthritis
Potassium	At least 4,000 milligrams	All meats, fish and vegetables Beet greens, prunes, soybeans, salmon, tomato paste, broccoli, sweet potato, bananas, blackstrap molasses	Restores balance to kidneys	High blood pressure Osteoporosis Kidney failure

WHAT TO AVOID	WHERE TO FIND IT	WHAT IT DOES	WHAT IT CAUSES
Omega-6 fat	Commercially-farmed meats & dairy Processed foods Bread and baked goods Vegetable oils (corn, soybean)	Promotes inflammation	Heart attack and stroke Alzheimer's disease Arthritis Asthma
Sugars and excess carbohydrate	Processed foods Sweets, desserts, candies Sweetened beverages Processed grains Dairy	Raises insulin levels	Diabetes Obesity Heart disease
Sodium	Processed foods, Baked goods Condiments Restaurant food Bottled beverages Soy sauce Smoked foods	Impairs kidney function	High blood pressure Kidney failure Osteoporosis Heart disease

By definition, the purpose of dietary supplements is to give you more of what you should already be getting in your diet. Now that you've done all the hard work of learning how to fill your plate with all-natural, nutrient-rich foods you can start clearing out a lot of unnecessary supplements and hopefully medications as well. That being said, there are a few supplements that I find myself suggesting to patients fairly often. This is hardly a comprehensive list but a good starting point for most people. Of course, be sure to discuss any supplements with your doctor before you begin taking them.

VITAMIN D

If you are following a healthy diet you shouldn't need a whole lot of vitamins since you'll get plenty in the food you are eating; however, the one vitamin you won't find in food is vitamin D. In fact, only oily fish like salmon and cod have any appreciable levels of vitamin D. We humans rely on the sun, not food, for our vitamin D, and unfortunately few people get enough to achieve healthy levels of this important vitamin.

Most people know that vitamin D is important for healthy bones, but few are aware of how far-reaching vitamin D's effects are. Vitamin D receptors are found throughout the body and affect nearly every part of healthy functioning. Studies show that vitamin D deficiency is associated with all of the following:

- Muscle weakness
- Higher risk of falls and fractures
- Heart disease and stroke
- Diabetes
- High cholesterol

- Colon, breast, and prostate cancers
- Multiple sclerosis
- Rheumatoid arthritis
- High blood pressure

Despite its myriad benefits, few people get enough vitamin D to see them. Even if you get plenty of sun compared to your peers, it is doubtful that you are getting enough to keep your vitamin D stores replete. Remember that our ancestors were out in the sun all day, every day, while we rarely get out for more than a few hours per week. Studies suggest that up to 95% of adults are vitamin D deficient, and even in San Diego these numbers aren't too far off. I'd say that about three-fourths of my patients on average are deficient in vitamin D without supplementation.

Vitamin D supplement doses range from a low of 400 to a high of 5,000 units (U) per pill. About 1,000 U daily is usually sufficient to achieve and maintain healthy blood levels of vitamin D, although more may be necessary in some cases. Vitamin D is fat-soluble, so taking it with food helps absorption.

A blood test for vitamin D is cheap and covered by most insurance plans. The optimal range is about 50–60 ng/mL, which is in the midpoint of the normal range. Luckily, vitamin D toxicity is rare and usually associated with exceptionally high doses approaching 10,000 U daily. Taking 1,000–2,000 U daily, or about 5,000–10,000 U per week on average, is likely to be a safe and effective dose.

FISH OIL

As we discussed in Challenge #2, fish oil is a great way to lower your total body inflammation along with your risk of heart disease and other inflammatory diseases. Ideally, you'd like to get your perfect omega-3 and omega-6 balance through diet; however, that can be difficult in today's world. All it takes is a few days a week of eating out and you're likely to swing toward an imbalance of omegas in your diet.

Fish oil supplementation is an easy way to ensure that you're getting your omega-3, no matter where your food came from. Fish oil consumption has been associated with a lower risk of heart disease and abnormal heart rhythms, reduced blood pressure and improved cholesterol, and improvement in many inflammatory diseases including arthritis and asthma. Furthermore, omega-3 supplementation is associated with a reduction in risk of both dementia and age-related eye diseases such as macular degeneration.

There is some concern that fish oils may be contaminated by toxins; however, this concern is unlikely to be warranted. A Consumer Labs report showed that among 35 tested fish oil supplements only two surpassed legal limits for PCBs, which are the most common contaminant. Interestingly, even though there are low levels of PCBs in virtually all fish oil supplements, the levels found in pills are actually far lower than those found in most store-bought fish. One study showed that a small serving of salmon contained about 17x more PCBs than the highest amount in any tested supplement. Mercury contamination, another common concern, is also unwarranted–reports indicate that mercury is rarely, if ever, found in fish oil supplements.

You are much more likely to die of heart disease than PCB poisoning, so I would put aside any reservations and start taking fish oil regularly. Aim for about 2-3 grams of omega-3s daily from diet and supplements.

RED YEAST RICE
An ancient Chinese secret to lowering your cholesterol

Red Yeast Rice is a fantastic example of a mundane food that turns out to have far-reaching medicinal properties. Red yeast rice has been a part of Asian diets since the Ming Dynasty in the 1300s. This simple dish, also used as a food coloring for its reddish hue, is prepared by fermenting yeast of the species *Monascus purpureus* over rice. The resulting reddish brown powder is what gives Peking duck, for example, its characteristic red veneer.

Records suggest that during the Ming Dynasty red yeast rice was already recognized for its health benefits as a medicinal food. It was specifically purported to improve circulation and chi, or energy force. Given that preventing heart attacks and strokes might be thought of as being consistent with good energy and good circulation, it seems those ancient Chinese were onto something even back then.

More recently, scientists in the 1970s discovered that the active compounds in red yeast rice, called "monacolins," were effective in lowering cholesterol. Monacolin K, the most promising of these compounds, was renamed "lovastatin" and patented as a prescription drug. Other drugs such as Lipitor, Zocor, and Crestor soon followed.

Red yeast rice preparations contain monacolin K (lovastatin) along with a host of other biologically similar compounds. A typical red yeast rice preparation contains a number of active ingredients including isoflavanes (similar to the active compounds in soy or chocolate), sterols, and nine monacolins, one of which is lovastatin.

LDL reductions of over 20% are achievable with 2.4 grams of red yeast rice daily (equivalent to only 5–7 milligrams of lovastatin), suggesting that the multiple active ingredients in red yeast rice confer a greater ability to lower cholesterol than would be implied by the amount of lovastatin alone. Not only does red yeast rice lower cholesterol, but large prospective randomized trials in China (where herbal medicines are given equal standing with pharmaceuticals) show that cardiovascular outcomes are similar to those of statins. For example, the China Coronary Secondary Prevention Study included over 5,000 patients and demonstrated that patients who received treatment with red yeast rice after a heart attack had a 45% reduction in coronary events, 62% reduction in non-fatal heart attacks, and 32% reduction in fatal heart attacks compared to those on placebo. These results rival those of statins in similar trials.

Unfortunately, you won't hear any of these results from the supplement companies because FDA regulations prohibit companies from promoting their products for cholesterol-lowering without running a clinical trial. As you might guess, few supplements companies have an interest in running a clinical trial for a natural product that can't be patented. Furthermore, since there is little oversight of the nutritional supplement industry, the quality of red yeast rice preparations tends to vary widely. The amount of monacolins (the active ingredients) in commercially available preparations of red yeast rice is very inconsistent, with some pills having zero active ingredients.

To make matters worse, the yeast fermentation process may yield a potentially toxic byproduct: citrinin. This toxin has been found in high concentrations in some preparations, particularly those with lower amounts of monacolins. Therefore, shopping blindly for red yeast rice products can be a risky proposition: you are either getting a lot of monacolins or a lot of toxin, and there's no way to know. Check out our website for more information on high-quality red yeast rice supplements.

If you have high cholesterol and are unwilling or unable to take a statin, it is worth considering red yeast rice. Data suggest that the side effect profile may be less than that of statins with respect to muscle aches, and the available studies suggest similar efficacy. As with any medication change, consult your doctor before switching to red yeast rice. You should definitely not take red yeast rice without consulting your doctor if you are currently taking medication for cholesterol.

PLANT STEROLS
A natural way to lower your cholesterol without medication

Plant sterols are the plant equivalent of the cholesterol found in animal tissue. These molecules have two significant health benefits relevant to most people: they lower cholesterol and they may reduce the risk of cancer.

The most common sterol used as a supplement is beta-sitosterol. Plant sterols like beta-sitosterol (and similar molecules called "stanols") look enough like cholesterol to bind to the cholesterol receptors in your intestinal tract. With your cholesterol receptors blocked by sterols, cholesterol will pass right through without being absorbed.

Beta-sitosterol   **Cholesterol**

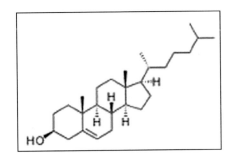

Can you tell the good twin from the evil twin?

A generally recommended dose of plant sterols for cholesterol reduction is at least 1,500 to 2,000 milligrams per day. This dose should be split up and taken before the 2 or 3 largest meals of the day. The largest amount of cholesterol is absorbed right after a fatty meal, especially one with animal fat that also has cholesterol.

Beta-sitosterol and its fellow sterols have also been shown to reduce the risk of certain cancers, including breast, colon, and prostate cancers, as well as to reduce the symptoms of benign prostate enlargement in men. The dose needed to accomplish these goals is around 60 milligrams per day, much less than that which is required to reduce cholesterol.

Sterols are found widely in extra virgin oils and fatty plants like nuts and avocados. A tablespoon of extra virgin olive oil contains about 30 milligrams of sterols or about half the cancer-preventing daily dose. An avocado has about 100 milligrams. You'll probably get enough sterols from your ancestral diet to reach the cancer-fighting, prostate-shrinking dose, but if you want to work on lowering your cholesterol, you're best served by using a dietary supplement.

SELECT BIBLIOGRAPHY

PART I: DIET, EXERCISE, SEE ME IN SIX MONTHS

National Health and Nutrition Examination Survey (NHANES).

US Dept. of Health and Human Services, CDC National Center for Health Statistics.

USDA National Nutrient Database for Standard Reference.

Katz, D. L. *Nutrition in Clinical Practice,* 2nd ed. Lippincott Williams & Wilkins, 2008.

Richards, M. P. "A brief review of the evidence for Paleolithic and Neolithic subsistence," *European Journal of Clinical Nutrition* (2002): 56.

Milton, K. "Micronutrient intakes of wild primates: are humans different?" *Comparative Biochemistry and Physiology* 136, no. 43 (2003): 47–59.

Milton, K. "Back to basics: why foods of wild primates have relevance for modern human health," *Nutrition* 16, no. 7/8 (2000): 480–483.

Nestle, M. "Animal v. plant foods in human diets and health: is the historical record unequivocal?" *Proceedings of the Nutrition Society* 58 (1999):211–218.

Milton, K. "Nutritional characteristics of wild primate foods: do the diets of our closest living relatives have lessons for us?" *Nutrition* 15, no. 6 (1999): 488–498.

Milton, K. "Hunter-gatherer diets–a different perspective," *American Journal of Clinical Nutrition* 71 (2000): 665–667.

Shoeninger, M. "The ancestral dinner table," *Nature* 487 (2012): 42–43.

Henry, A. "The diet of *Australopithecus sediba*," *Nature* 487 (2012): 90–93.

Cordain, L. "Plant-animal subsistence ratios and macronutrient energy estimations in worldwide hunter-gatherer diets," *American Journal of Clinical Nutrition* 71 (2000): 682–92.

Cordain, L. "Origins and evolution of the Western diet: health implications for the 21st century," *American Journal of Clinical Nutrition* 81 (2005): 341–54.

Konner, M. "Paleolithic nutrition. A consideration of its nature and current implications," *New England Journal of Medicine* 315, no. 5 (1985): 283–289.

Konner, M. "Paleolithic nutrition, 25 years later," *Nutrition in Clinical Practice* 25, no. 6 (2010): 594–602.

Fiorenza, L. "Molar macrowear reveals Neanderthal eco-geographic dietary variation," *PLOS ONE* 6, no. 3 (2011): e14769.

Pijl, H. "Obesity: evolution of a symptom of affluence. How food has shaped our existence," *Netherlands Journal of Medicine* 69, no. 4 (2011).

Milton, K. "A hypothesis to explain the role of meat-eating in human evolution," *Evolutionary Anthropology* 8, no. 1 (1999): 11–21.

National Cattlemen's Beef Association.

Daley, C. "A review of fatty acid profiles and antioxidant content in grass-fed and grain-fed beef." *Nutrition Journal* 9, no. 10 (2010).

Leheska, J. M. "Effects of conventional and grass-feeding systems on the nutrient composition of beef," *Journal of Animal Science* 86 (2008): 3575–3585.

Segers, J. R. "Effect of long-term corn by-product feeding on beef quality, strip loin fatty acid profiles, and shelf life," *Journal of Animal Science* 89 (2011): 3792– 3802.

Gebauer, S. K. "Effects of Ruminant trans-Fatty Acids on Cardiovascular Disease and Cancer: A Comprehensive Review of Epidemiological, Clinical, and Mechanistic Studies," *Advanced Nutrition* 2 (2011): 332–354.

Luciano, G. "Vitamin E and polyunsaturated fatty acids in bovine muscle and the oxidative stability of beef from cattle receiving grass or concentrate-based rations," *Journal of Animal Science* 89 (2011): 3759–3768.

Koeth, R. "Intestinal microbiota metabolism of L-carnitine, a nutrient in red meat, promotes atherosclerosis," *National Medicine* 19, no. 5 (2013): 576–585.

Wang, Z. "Gut flora metabolism of phosphatidylcholine promotes cardiovascular disease," *Nature* 472, no. 7341 (2011): 57–63.

Tang, W. H. "Intestinal microbial metabolism of phosphatidylcholine and cardio-vascular risk," *New England Journal of Medicine* 368, no. 17 (2013): 1575–1584.

Loscalzo, J. "Gut microbiota, the genome, and diet in atherogenesis," *New England Journal of Medicine* 368, no. 17 (2013): 1647–1649.

Nijeboer, P. "Non-celiac gluten sensitivity. Is it in the gluten or the grain?" *Journal of Gastrointestinal and Liver Diseases* 22, no. 4 (2013): 435–440.

Dodd, H. "Calculating meal glycemic index by using measured and published food values compared with directly measured meal glycemic index," *American Journal of Clinical Nutrition* 94, no. 992 (2011): 992–996.

Chakravarthy, M. "Eating, exercise, and 'thrifty' genotypes: connecting the dots toward an evolutionary understanding of modern chronic diseases," *Journal of Applied Physiology* 96 (2004): 3–10.

Mann, J. "Diet and diabetes revisited, yet again," *American Journal of Clinical Nutrition* 97 (2013): 453–454.

Tzagournis, M. "Triglycerides in clinical medicine, a review," American Journal of Clinical Nutrition 31 (1978): 1437–1452.

Rong, Y. "Egg consumption and risk of coronary heart disease and stroke: dose-response meta-analysis of prospective cohort studies," *BMJ* (2013): 346.

Liener, I. "Toxic Factors in Edible Legumes and Their Elimination," *American Journal of Clinical Nutrition* 11 (Oct. 1962).

Messina, M. J. "Legumes and soybeans: overview of their nutritional profiles and health effects." *American Journal of Clinical Nutrition* 70, supplement (1999): 439S–450S.

Dahl, W. "Review of the Health Benefits of Peas," *British Journal of Nutrition* 108, supplement (2012): S3–S10.

Story, J. "Interactions of alfalfa plant and sprout Saponins with cholesterol in vitro and in cholesterol-fed rats," *American Journal of Clinical Nutrition* 39 (1984): 917–929.

Rao, A. V. "Saponins as anticarcinogens," *Journal of Nutrition* 125 (1995): 7178–7248.

Tsa, C. "Effect of soy saponin on the growth of human colon cancer cells," *World Journal of Gastroenterology* 16, no. 27 (2010): 3371–3376.

Johnson, I. T. "Influence of Saponins on gut permeability and active nutrient transport in vitro," *Journal of Nutrition* 166 (1986): 2270–2277.

Lam, S. "Lectins: production and practical applications," *Applied Microbiology and Biotechnology* 89 (2011): 45–55.

Nachbar, M. "Lectins in the United States diet: a survey of lectins in commonly consumed foods and a review of the literature," *American Journal of Clinical Nutrition* 33 (1980): 2338–2345.

Simopoulos, A. "N-3 fatty acids in eggs from range-fed Greek chickens," *New England Journal of Medicine* 321 (1989): 1412.

Etherton, K. "Nuts and their bioactive constituents: effects on serum lipids and other factors that affect disease risk." *American Journal of Clinical Nutrition* 70, supplement (1999): 504S–511S.

Etherton, K. "The role of tree nuts and peanuts in the prevention of coronary heart disease: multiple potential mechanisms," *Journal of Nutrition* 138, supplement (2008): 1746S–1751S.

Mukuddem-Petersen, J. "A systematic review of the effects of nuts on blood lipid profiles in humans," *Journal of Nutrition* 135 (2005): 2082–2089.

Andrikopoulos, N. K. "Deterioration of natural antioxidant species of vegetable edible oils during the domestic deep-frying and pan-frying of potatoes," *International Journal of Food Sciences and Nutrition* 53 (2002): 351–363.

Estruch, R. "Primary prevention of cardiovascular disease with a Mediterranean diet," *New England Journal of Medicine* 368 (2013): 1279-1290.

Farshchi, H. "Deleterious effects of omitting breakfast on insulin sensitivity and fasting lipid profiles in healthy lean women," *American Journal of Clinical Nutrition* 81 (2005): 388–396.

PART III: THE CHALLENGES
CHALLENGE #2: GET FAT!

Katan, M. "Effects of fats and fatty acids on blood lipids in humans: an overview," *American Journal of Clinical Nutrition* 60, supplement (1994): 1017S–1022S.

Lipoeto, N. "Dietary intake and the risk of coronary heart disease among the coconut-consuming Minangkabau in West Sumatra, Indonesia," *Asia Pacific Journal of Clinical Nutrition* 13, no. 4 (2004): 377–384.

Barona, J. "Dietary Cholesterol Affects Plasma Lipid Levels, the Intravascular Processing of Lipoproteins and Reverse Cholesterol Transport without Increasing the Risk for Heart Disease," *Nutrients* 4 (2012): 1015–1025.

Chen, B. "Multi-country analysis of palm oil consumption and cardiovascular disease mortality for countries at different stages of economic development: 1980–1997," *Globalization and Health* 7 (2011): 45.

Voon, P. "Diets high in palmitic acid (16:0), lauric and myristic acids (12:0 + 14:0), or oleic acid (18:1) do not alter postprandial or fasting plasma homocysteine and inflammatory markers in healthy Malaysian adults," *American Journal of Clinical Nutrition* 94 (2011): 1451–1457.

Barona, J. "Coconut oil predicts a beneficial lipid profile in pre-menopausal women in the Philippines," *Nutrients* 4 (2012): 1015–1025.

Lawrence, G. "Dietary Fats and Health: Dietary Recommendations in the Context of Scientific Evidence," *Advances in Nutrition* 4 (2013): 294–302.

Astrup, A. "The role of reducing intakes of saturated fat in the prevention of cardiovascular disease: where does the evidence stand in 2010?" *American Journal of Clinical Nutrition* 93 (2011): 684–688.

Stephenson, J. "The Multifaceted Effects of Omega-3 Polyunsaturated Fatty Acids on the Hallmarks of Cancer," *Journal of Lipids* (2013).

Ailhaud, G. "Temporal changes in dietary fats: role of n-6 polyunsaturated fatty acids in excessive adipose tissue development and relationship to obesity," *Progress in Lipid Research* (Feb. 2006): 203–236.

Patterson, E. "Health Implications of High Dietary Omega-6 Polyunsaturated Fatty Acids," *Journal of Nutrition and Metabolism* (2012).

Chan, E. "What can we expect from omega-3 fatty acids?" *Cleveland Clinic Journal of Medicine* 76, no. 4 (2009).

Ho, K. "Alaskan arctic Eskimo: responses to a customary high fat diet," American Journal of Clinical Nutrition 25 (1972): 737–745.

Yamagishi, K. "Dietary intake of saturated fatty acids and incident stroke and coronary heart disease in Japanese communities," *European Heart Journal* 34, no. 16 (2013): 1225–1232.

Barona, J. "Dietary cholesterol affects plasma lipid levels, the intravascular processing of lipoproteins and reverse cholesterol transport without increasing the risk for heart disease," *Nutrients* 4 (2012): 1015–1025.

Soelaiman, I. "Serum lipids, lipid peroxidation and glutathione peroxidase activity in rats on long-term feeding with coconut oil or butterfat (ghee)," *Asia Pacific Journal of Clinical Nutrition* 5, no. 4 (1996): 244–248.

Massiera, F. "A Western-like fat diet is sufficient to induce a gradual enhancement in fat mass over generations," *Journal of Lipid Research* 51 (2010).

Jungheim, E. "Obesity and reproductive function," *Obstetrics & Gynecology Clinics of North America* 39 (2012): 479–493.

Palmer, N. "Impact of obesity on male fertility, sperm function and molecular composition," *Spermatogenesis* 2, no. 4 (2012): 253–263.

CHALLENGE #3: PLEASE DON'T PASS THE SALT

Forbes, G. "Total sodium, potassium and chloride in adult man," *Journal of Clinical Investigation* 35, no. 6 (1956): 596–600.

Kotchen, T. "Salt in health and disease—a delicate balance," *New England of Journal of Medicine* 368 (2013): 1229–1237.

Staessen, J. "Salt and blood pressure in community-based intervention trials," *American Journal of Clinical Nutrition* 65, supplement (1997): 661S–670S.

Cutler, J. "Randomized trials of sodium reduction: an overview," *American Journal of Clinical Nutrition* 65, supplement (1997): 643S–651S.

INTERSALT Cooperative Research Group. "INTERSALT: An international study of electrolyte excretion and blood pressure. Results for 24-hour urinary sodium and potassium excretion," *BMJ* 297 (1988): 319–330.

Stamler, J. "The INTERSALT Trial: Background, methods, findings, and implications," *American Journal of Clinical Nutrition* 65, supplement (1997): 626S–642S.

Carvalho, M. J. "Blood pressure in four remote populations in the INTERSALT study," *Hypertension* 14 (1989): 238–246.

Frassetto, LA. "Dietary sodium chloride intake independently predicts the degree of hyperchloremic metabolic acidosis in healthy humans consuming a net acid-producing diet," *American Journal of Physiology – Renal Physiology* 293 (2007): F521–F525.

Lim, S. "Metabolic acidosis," *Acta Medica Indonesiana – Indonesian Journal of Internal Medicine* 39, no. 3 (2007): 145–150.

Golembiewska, E. "Renal tubular acidosis—underrated problem?" *Acta Biochimica Polonica* 59 (2012): 213–217.

Cogswell, M. "Sodium and potassium intakes among US adults: NHANES 2003-2008," *American Journal of Clinical Nutrition* 96 (2012): 647–657.

Sellmeyer, D. "A high ratio of dietary animal to vegetable protein increases the rate of bone loss and the risk of fracture in postmenopausal women," *American Journal of Clinical Nutrition* 73 (2001): 118–122.

Heaney, R. "Protein intake and bone health: the influence of belief systems on the conduct of nutritional science," *American Journal of Clinical Nutrition* 73 (2001): 5–6.

Macdonald, H. "Low dietary potassium intakes and high dietary estimates of net endogenous acid production are associated with low bone mineral density in premenopausal women and increased markers of bone resorption in post-menopausal women," *American Journal of Clinical Nutrition* 81 (2005): 923–933.

Strohle, A. "Estimation of the diet-dependent net acid load in 229 worldwide historically studied hunter-gatherer societies," *American Journal of Clinical Nutrition* 91 (2010): 406–412.

Sebastian, A. "Estimation of the net acid load of the diet of ancestral pre-agricultural *homo sapiens* and their hominid ancestors," *American Journal of Clinical Nutrition* 76 (2002): 1308–1316.

Camien, M. "A critical reappraisal of 'acid-base' balance," *American Journal of Clinical Nutrition* 22, no. 6 (1969): 786–793.

Fraunhofer, J. "Dissolution of dental enamel in soft drinks," *Academy of General Dentistry* (2004): 308–312.

Sebastian, A. "Improved mineral balance and skeletal metabolism in postmenopausal women treated with potassium bicarbonate," *New England Journal of Medicine* 330 (1994): 1776–1781.

Jacobson, M. "Changes in sodium levels in processed and restaurant foods, 2005–2011," *JAMA Internal Medicine* 173, no. 14 (2013): 1285–1291.

Mattes, R. "The taste for salt in humans," *American Journal of Clinical Nutrition* 65, supplement (1997): 692S–697S.

Samelson, E. "Calcium intake is not associated with increased coronary artery calcification: the Framingham Study," *American Journal of Clinical Nutrition* 96 (2012): 1274–1280.

Reid, I. "Cardiovascular effects of calcium supplements," *Nutrients* 5 (2013): 2522–2529.

Prentice, R. L. "Health risks and benefits from calcium and vitamin D supplementation: Women's Health Initiative clinical trial and cohort study," *Osteoporosis International* 24 (2013): 567–580.

Jamal, S. "Calcium builds strong bones, and more is better–correct? Well, maybe not," *Clinical Journal of the American Society of Nephrology* 7 (2012): 1877–1883.

CHALLENGE #4: FIBER

Bosscher, D. "Food-based strategies to modulate the composition of the intestinal microbiota and their associated health effects," Journal of Physiology and Pharmacology 60, supplement 6, (2009): S5–S11.

Streppel, M. "Dietary fiber intake in relation to coronary heart disease and all-cause mortality over 40 y: the Zutphen Study," *American Journal of Clinical Nutrition* 88 (2008): 1119–1125.

Delzenne, N. "Modulation of the gut microbiota by nutrients with prebiotic properties: consequences for host health in the context of obesity and metabolic syndrome," *Microbial Cell Factories* 10, supplement (2011): S10.

Higgins, P. "Epidemiology of constipation in North America: a systematic review," *American Journal of Gastroenterology* (2004): 750–759.

Milton, K. "Digestion and passage kinetics of chimpanzees fed high and low fiber diets and comparison with human data," *Journal of Nutrition* 118 (1988): 1082–1088.

Anderson, J. "Health benefits and practical aspects of high fiber diets," *American Journal of Clinical Nutrition* 59, supplement (1994): 1242S–1247S.

Boeing, H. "Critical review: vegetables and fruit in the prevention of chronic diseases," *European Journal of Nutrition* 51 (2012): 637–663.

Sanchez, M. "Epidemiology and burden of chronic constipation," *Canadian Journal of Gastroenterology* 25, supplement B (2011): 11B–15B.

Weikert, M. "Metabolic effects of dietary fiber consumption and prevention of diabetes," *Journal of Nutrition* 138 (2008): 439s–442.

Kaczmarczyk, M. "The health benefits of dietary fiber: beyond the usual suspects of type 2 diabetes, cardiovascular disease and colon cancer," *Metabolism* 61, no. 8 (2012): 1058–1066.

Lohsiriwat, V. "Hemorrhoids: from basic pathophysiology to clinical management," *World Journal of Gastroenterology* 18, no. 17 (2012): 2009–2017.

Samra, R. "Insoluble cereal fiber reduces appetite and short-term food intake and glycemic response to food consumed 75 min later by healthy men," *American Journal of Clinical Nutrition* 86 (2007): 972–979.

Davis, C. "Gastrointestinal microflora, food components and colon cancer prevention," *Journal of Nutritional Biochemistry* 20, no. 10 (2009): 743–752.

Lattimer, J. "Effects of dietary fiber and its components on metabolic health," *Nutrients* 2 (2010): 1266–1289.

Slavin, J. "Fiber and prebiotics: mechanisms and health benefits," *Nutrients* 5 (2013): 1417–1435.

Grooms, K. "Dietary fiber intake and cardiometabolic risks among US adults, NHANES 1999-2010," *American Journal of Medicine* 126 (2013): 1059-1067.

Haggar, F. "Colorectal cancer epidemiology: incidence, mortality, survival and risk factors," *Clinics in Colon and Rectal Surgery* 22, no. 4 (2009): 191-197.

CHALLENGE #5: ANTIOXIDANTS

USDA Database for the isoflavone content of selected foods, release 2.0.

Ribaric, S. "Diet and Aging," *Oxidative Medicine and Cellular Longevity* (2012).

Ergin, V. "Carbonyl stress in aging process: role of vitamins and phytochemicals as redox regulators," *Aging and Disease* 4, no. 5 (2013): 276-294.

Gutowski, M. "A study of free radical chemistry: their role and pathophysiological significance," *Acta Biochimica Polonica* 60, no. 1 (2013): 1-16.

Halvorsen, B. "Content of redox-active compounds (i.e., antioxidants) in foods consumed in the United States," *American Journal of Clinical Nutrition* 84 (2006): 95-135.

Lambert, J. "Inhibition of carcinogenesis by polyphenols: evidence from laboratory investigations," *American Journal of Clinical Nutrition* 81, supplement (2005): 284S-291S.

Nijveldt, R. "Flavonoids: a review of probable mechanisms of action and potential applications," *American Journal of Clinical Nutrition* 74 (2001): 418-425.

Kizhakekuttu, T. J. "Natural Antioxidants and Hypertension: Promise and Challenges," *Cardiovascular Therapeutics* 28, no. 4 (2010): e20-e32.

Hammond, B. R. "Carotenoids," *Advances in Nutrition* 4 (2013): 474-476.

Aslam, T. "Micronutrients in age-related macular degeneration," *Ophthalmologica* 229 (2013): 75–79.

AREDS2 Research Group. "Lutein + zeaxanthin and omega-3 fatty acids for age-related macular degeneration. The AREDS2 randomized clinical trial," *Journal of the American Medical Association* 309, no. 19 (2013): 2005–15.

Seddon, J. "Dietary carotenoids, vitamins A, C, and E, and advanced age-related macular degeneration," *Journal of the American Medical Association* 272, no. 18 (1994): 1413–1420.

Jarrett, S. "Consequences of oxidative stress in age-related macular degeneration," *Molecular Aspects of Medicine* 33, no. 4 (2012): 399–417.

Bone, R. "Lutein and zeaxanthin dietary supplements raise macular pigment density and serum concentrations of these carotenoids in humans," *Journal of Nutrition* 133 (2003): 992–998.

Arab, L. "Lycopene and cardiovascular disease," *American Journal of Clinical Nutrition* 71, supplement (2000): 1691S–1695S.

Story, E. "An update on the health effects of tomato lycopene," *Annual Review of Food Science and Technology* 1 (2010).

Wang, X. "Lycopene metabolism and its biological significance," *American Journal of Clinical Nutrition* 96, supplement (2012): 1214S–1222S.

Patisaul, H. "The pros and cons of phytoestrogens," *Frontiers in Neuroendocrinology* 31, no. 4 (2010): 400–419.

Messina, M. "A brief historical overview of the past two decades of soy and isoflavone research," *Journal of Nutrition* 140 (2010): 1350S–1354S.

Deibert, P. "Soy protein based supplementation supports metabolic effects of resistance training in previously untrained middle aged males," *Aging Male* 14, no. 4 (2011): 273–279.

Jurenka, J. "Anti-inflammatory properties of curcumin, a major constituent of curcumina longa: a review of clinical and preclinical research," *Alternative Medicine Review* 14, no. 2 (2009): 141–153.

Mishra, S. "The effect of curcumin on Alzheimer's disease: an overview," *Annals of Indian Academy of Neurology* 11, no. 1 (2008): 13–19.

Ganguli, M. "Apolipoprotein E polymorphism and Alzheimer disease. The Indo-US Cross-National Dementia Study," *Archives of Neurology* 57 (2000): 824– 830.

Ng, T-P. "Curry consumption and cognitive function in the elderly," *American Journal of Epidemiology* 164, no. 9 (2006): 898–906.

Mukhtar, H. "Tea polyphenols: prevention of cancer and optimizing health," *American Journal of Clinical Nutrition* 71, supplement (2000): 1698S–1702S.

Dwyer, J. "Tea and flavonoids: where we are, where to go next," *American Journal of Clinical Nutrition* 98, supplement (2013): 1611S–1618S.

Arab, L. "Tea consumption and cardiovascular risk," *American Journal of Clinical Nutrition* 98, supplement (2013): 1651S–1659S.

Yuan, J. "Cancer prevention by green tea: evidence from epidemiologic studies," *American Journal of Clinical Nutrition* 98, supplement (2013): 1676S–1681S.

Yang, D. J. "Effects of different steeping methods and storage on caffeine, catechins and gallic acid in bag tea infusions," *Journal of Chromatography A* 1156, no. 1–2 (2007): 312–320.

Weiss, D. "Determination of catechins in matcha green tea by micellar electrokinetic chromatography," *Journal of Chromatography A* 1011, no. 1–2 (2003): 173–180.

Nigdikar, S. "Consumption of red wine polyphenols reduces the susceptibility of low-density lipoproteins to oxidation in vivo," *American Journal of Clinical Nutrition* 68 (1998): 258–265.

Waterhouse, A. "Is it time for a wine trial?" *American Journal of Clinical Nutrition* 68 (1998): 220–221.

Renaud, S. "Moderate wine drinkers have lower hypertension-related mortality: a prospective cohort study in French men," *American Journal of Clinical Nutrition* 80 (2004): 621–625.

Chung, J. "Resveratrol as a calorie restriction mimetic: therapeutic implications," *Trends in Cell Biology* 22, no. 10 (2012): 546–554.

Miller, K. "Survey of commercially available chocolate- and cocoa-containing products in the United States. Comparison of flavan-3-ol content with nonfat cocoa solids, total polyphenols, and percent cacao," *Journal of Agricultural and Food Chemistry* 57 (2009): 9169–9180.

Miller, K. "Antioxidant activity and polyphenol and procyanidin contents of selected commercially available cocoa-containing and chocolate products in the United States," *Journal of Agricultural and Food Chemistry* 54, no. 11 (2006): 4062–4068.

Payne, M. J. "Impact of fermentation, drying, roasting and Dutch processing on epicatechin and catechin content of cacao beans and cocoa ingredients," *Journal of Agricultural and Food Chemistry* 58, no. 19 (2010): 10518–10527.

Andujar, I. "Cocoa Polyphenols and Their Potential Benefits for Human Health," *Oxidative Medicine and Cellular Longevity* (2012).

Hooper, L. "Effects of chocolate, cocoa, and flavan-3-ols on cardiovascular health: a systematic review and meta-analysis of randomized trials," *American Journal of Clinical Nutrition* 95 (2012): 740–751.

Reid, C. "The effectiveness and cost effectiveness of dark chocolate consumption as prevention therapy in people at high risk of cardiovascular disease: best case scenario analysis using a Markov model," *BMJ* 344 (2012): e3657.

SUPPLEMENTS

Holick, M. "The vitamin D epidemic and its health consequences," *Journal of Nutrition* 135, supplement (2005): 2739S–2748S.

Ware, W. "The JUPITER lipid lowering trial and vitamin D. Is there a connection?" *Dermato-Endocrinology* 2, no. 2 (2010): 50–54.

Makariou, S. "The relationship of vitamin D with non-traditional risk factors for cardiovascular disease in subjects with metabolic syndrome," *Archives of Medical Science* 8, no. 3 (2012): 437–443.

Zhang, R. "Vitamin D in health and disease: current perspectives," *Nutrition Journal* 9 (2010): 65.

Wang, H. "Influence of vitamin D supplementation on plasma lipid profiles: a meta-analysis of randomized controlled trials," *Lipids in Health and Disease* 11 (2012): 42.

Russell, F. "Distinguishing health benefits of eicosapentaenoic acid and docosahexaenoic acids," *Marine Drugs* 10 (2012): 2535–2559.

Becker, D. J. "Simvastatin vs therapeutic lifestyle changes and supplements: randomized primary prevention trial," *Mayo Clinic Proceedings* 83, no. 7 (2008): 758–764.

Carter, M. "Is Red Yeast Rice a Suitable Alternative for Statins?" *Mayo Clinic Proceedings* 83, no. 11 (2008): 1294–1301.

Gordon, R. "Marked Variability of Monacolin Levels in Commercial Red Yeast Rice Products, Buyer Beware!" *Archives of Internal Medicine* 170, no. 19 (2010): 1722–1727.

Becker, D. J. "Red Yeast Rice for Dyslipidemia in Statin-Intolerant Patients A Randomized Trial," *Annals of Internal Medicine* 150 (2009): 830–839.

Awad, A. "Phytosterols as Anticancer Dietary Components: Evidence and Mechanism of Action," *Journal of Nutrition* 130 (2000): 2127–2130.

Scholle, J. "The effect of adding plant sterols or stanols to statin therapy in hyper-cholesterolemic patients: systematic review and meta-analysis," *Journal of the American College of Nutrition* 28, no. 5 (2009): 517–524.

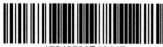

Made in the USA
San Bernardino, CA
11 December 2014